# 34 Sleeve Patient Stories

## The *Real Truth* About Gastric Sleeve Surgery in Mexico

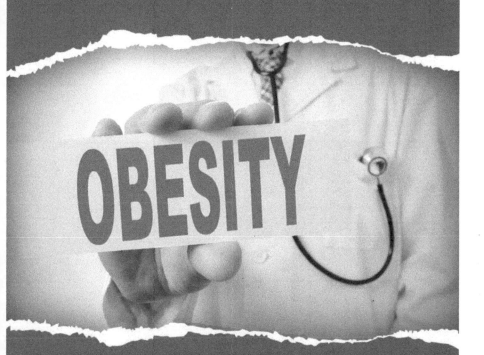

ISBN: 978-1502464538

www.thegastricsleeve.com

Printed and bound in the United States of America

Published by MBM Publishing
4000 East Bristol Street, Suite 3
Elkhart, IN 46514

# INTRODUCTION

Throughout the years I've had thousands of patients that come mainly from the United States and Canada to our weight loss surgery center but we've also received patients from every continent in the world. Our goal is to have a top-notch facility, be always accessible to patients and offer them high-quality healthcare for half the price found in the United States.

I know that for most of these patients that have crossed the border it has come to their minds "What am I doing coming to Mexico?, Will I be safe? Will everything be alright?, etc."

Believe me that throughout these years I think I've hear it all.

At one point some years ago, I even had this lady ask me if she would still have her kidneys when she woke up! In a sarcastic way I replied that unfortunately we couldn't remove any of her organs through the tiny incisions that we do when performing a gastric sleeve surgery.

That was many years ago.

Nowadays we fortunately have the internet to help us have more confidence on what we do, what we buy and what services are reliable. Today's tools, like Facebook, put us directly with patients that have previously gone through this procedure and with a surgical team which you can interact with them and have an idea of what to expect.

YouTube, for example, is another great tool to be able to see facilities, your doctor and your surgical team and be in contact with valuable information from your surgeon's practice.

I could name many other tools like twitter, Google+, forums, podcasts, Pinterest, etc. that have made everything so transparent that you literally know how everything is and what the experience will be like with choosing a surgical practice. I know all this because I personally use these tools to help my patients feel comfortable, to let them know that I'm always available to them and that we are a team that will back you up always.

My patients know this and they know that we are just a click away. Social media has changed the rules of practically everything, including medicine but nothing, nothing ever beats one thing: "Word of mouth".

I believe that like in any business your work speaks out for itself.

So I've put together a series of stories that I know you'll enjoy reading. I know you'll learn from my patients and you'll get to see the real story behind the gastric sleeve and the real story about going to another country (even though it's just 1 mile from the border) for their gastric sleeve procedure.

These stories have been sent by my patients and are unedited so you'll read it as it is. I know you'll enjoy them as much as I did as they were being submitted by my patients. If you are interested in reading more stories, testimonials, watching photos and videos you can always visit my website www.endobariatric.com.

Finally I would like to thank all my patients for their support in helping me put this book together. I'm very grateful to each and one of you who took the time to send your stories, pictures and be willing to help future patients who are struggling with obesity. I know these stories share with us the transformation, the success and the experience having a sleeve gastrectomy but my patients need to understand that they too are changing people's lives by doing this.

We are a community, a weight loss surgery community and we should always lend each other a hand. Words cannot express the immense gratitude I have toward my patients for helping me do this.

Enjoy!

Guillermo Alvarez, M.D.
Piedras Negras, Mexico
866-697-5338
www.Endobariatric.com

# TABLE OF CONTENTS

# MOSTLY A RECLUSE

**Tessa B.** - My sleeve journey began in December of

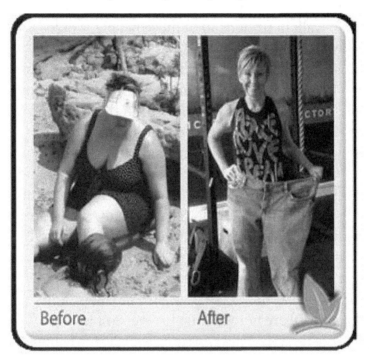

Before            After

2010 when a family member was talking at the
dinner table about a friend who went to Mexico and
had most of her stomach removed to lose weight. At
that point in my life, I was mostly a recluse. I was
mentally, physically, and emotionally exhausted and
in pain. I was on meds for depression, muscle pain,
undergoing tests for MS and other symptoms, having
breathing problems, and the list goes on. Nothing
was ever confirmed other than depression. That was
3 ½ years and 110 lbs ago. I now understand what
obesity is and how it was completely consuming me.

It's not just a number on the scale, a BMI number, a certain size clothes. It's a lot of things to me. I wouldn't leave the house because I didn't want people to see me, would sit on the closest bleacher to the entrance when going to a game because I didn't want to walk in front of all of those people, would quickly buy clothes at a store and not try them on because it was embarrassing and exhausting to try to find a fit or seen in the Plus sizes. My maternity jeans were my favorite pants to wear .- even three years after the birth of my daughter! I didn't have the energy nor the breath to do ordinary things. I had given up and watched so many opportunities pass me by due to my lack of confidence, poor self-esteem and bad health. I was miserable. That night at the dinner table in 2010, I found hope. If I had been diagnosed with a heart condition, lung disease, or MS, there would have been no question as to finding treatment. But obesity was the issue. Diet pills, fad diets, and diet centers were not working for me. So I took a more drastic step – the gastric sleeve. Surely I should be just as aggressive to battle obesity, which can lead to other diseases, so I did it. I made the decision to have sleeve surgery. I called my friend who had surgery in November, asked lots of questions, she gave me Dr. Alvarez's book, and I called Susan. Within the week I had my surgery date for January 10, 2011. From the first time I had contact with Susan and to this day, she has been an incredible source of support and reassurance. Dr. Alvarez and his team (including Rosie) were wonderful.

My surgery was short and sweet, no complications, and I was amazed at how well I felt afterwards. I'm sure you have heard many wonderful experiences from patients of Dr. Alvarez...mine is no exception.

Dr. Alvarez is not only best surgeon, he is also a great man. He continues to have contact with patients, provides motivation and encouragement through his radio show and social media, and genuinely cares about those who battle obesity.

My life has changed tremendously since my sleeve surgery – I no longer sit aside and watch life pass me by. I live it. I have a healthy relationship with food for the first time since being a teenager. I don't obsess about counting calories, fats, etc. I listen to my sleeve, eat protein and natural foods first, maybe a dessert every now and then and try to balance everything. I work out for 45 minutes 3 days per week with weights and interval training. I have never been a runner, but ran/walked my first half marathon in November of 2011 and continue to run 1 per year. It reminds me of where I have been and how far I have come.

Some people worry about not losing weight as fast as others. I am 3 years out and have finally found my happy place. It took me three years. I lost 80lbs the first year and have gradually lost the last 30lbs over the next 2 years, going from a size 24W to a 4.

My body continues to change, especially with consistent exercise. My actual weight has gone up since beginning weight training but my clothing size has gone down. I won't lie, I didn't like the lose skin on my hips when I ran or while wearing a swimming suit, so I had a lower body lift this past November. It was the icing on the cake.

I'm happy, I'm healthy and I love where I am with myself.

I no longer hide, I treat myself a lot better, and can finally look in the mirror and see someone I like, someone healthy, someone strong. Thank you so much Dr. Alvarez, Susan, the Endobariatric team, and my sleeve family. You all have been and continue to be a blessing. I'm forever grateful for each and every one of you. Love, Tess

# COULDN'T GO FOR WALKS ANYMORE

**Nancy R.** - I would recommend Dr. Alvarez to anyone who is thinking about weight loss surgery. My experience with him has been outstanding. From start to finish, everything was seamless!

Dr. A has thought of everything.

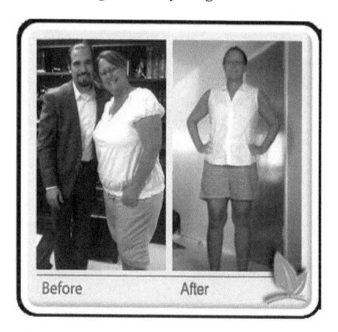

Before        After

Going to Mexico was a bit of a concern for me at first, but after reading and watching all the testimonials on his website, and those on YouTube, my mind was put to ease. And from my experience I have to tell you, I got better care from Dr. Alvarez and his staff than I have in the USA. My recovery has gone very well, and any questions I have are in the written information I have, or Susan or Dr. Alvarez are there to answer them. My surgery date was August 1, 2013. I am 4 weeks post-op and I have lost 34 lbs. since the beginning of my pre-op liquid diet, and 21 lbs. since surgery. Most of all I am active again!! The main reason I had surgery was because I couldn't go for walks anymore because of back pain. I am now walking and going to aqua class and loving it! Dr. Alvarez changed my life, and I will always be eternally grateful!!

# REQUIRED 4 WEEK LIQUID DIET

January 2013          March 2014

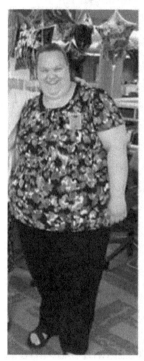 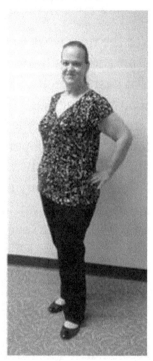

**Kandice P.** - Dr. Alvarez has assembled an amazing team. He and his entire team, Susan, Rosy, Andrea, Jessica, Dr. Gabe, Dr. Rosales & Dr. Salinas all have the same passion for helping people fighting obesity as he does. On May 20, 2013 I sent a message to info@endobatric.com to learn more about Vertical Sleeve Gastrectomy.

Within a day maybe less, Susan responded to me answering my questions as well as sending a video with Dr. Alvarez explaining what the procedure is all about. With this knowledge and all the information I researched online plus all the video Dr. Alvarez has online, I knew this was the right decision for me.

Over the next week or so I had a lot of questions for Susan and she always answered them promptly. She has a vast amount of knowledge about this procedure because she has also been a patient. She can also give you a personal perspective. Once I filled out all the Medical History paperwork and submitted it for approval it was only a matter of a few days before Dr. Alvarez reviewed my medical history and I was approved. I knew my journey was starting and I was looking forward to every minute of it.

I was a larger person when I started so I was required to complete a 4 week liquid diet (you may think 4 weeks - Oh my gosh but I knew I could do it.) My surgery was set for exactly 2 months later. I decided to start cutting back at that point; I didn't want to have a last meal, or food funeral. I decided at that point I wanted my liver and other organs to be in the best health they could be in for surgery. I started drinking 2 protein shakes and one small protein rich meal for dinner a day for the first month, and really didn't have any carb withdrawal headaches. In 4 weeks I had lost 25 lbs. I couldn't believe it. I thought to myself.. Maybe I can do this. This gave me the encouragement I need to keep going.

Now I was 4 weeks out from Surgery and my all liquid diet started. I replace my 3rd meal a day with one more shake (with lots of research and watching a lot of you-tube videos from other VSG people, I learned Premiere Protein is the best).

Finally the weekend before my surgery arrived. I made it... My mom decided to come with me to Piedras Negras, MX. We live in the Pacific Northwest and had to travel a day early in order to meet Rosy at the Hotel on Sunday morning for our 2.5 hour drive to Eagle Pass.

Rosy is wonderful; she has this process down to a science, and knew exactly where to stop for a break and explained things that we were seeing as we are driving to Eagle Pass. If I remember correctly she has been a part of Dr. Alvarez team for over 7 years. We arrived at the Holiday inn Express around 2:30 pm and Rosy checked us into the Hotel, she then told us that she would be back at around 7:00 am the next morning (Surgery Day).

Just like clockwork she met us at 7:00 am and drove us across the border into Mexico. Within a few minutes we were pulling into the parking lot of the Dr. Alvarez's office and were unloading our luggage.

When we walked into the office, Dr. Alvarez and Andrea both greeted us. We all sat down for a couple minutes and chatted with the Dr. Alvarez, he put us all at ease. When it was my turn to meet with Dr. Alvarez in his office I was weighed (and had lost a total of 50 lbs lost prior to surgery), a few pictures were taken and he discussed what was going to happen. He also answered any questions I had.

Andrea collected all our paperwork and took us next door from his office to the small private hospital. Then I started surgery prep, having blood drawn and a chest x-ray done, Andrea was with me every step of the way. Once back in my room I changed into my gown and waited a few minutes for the nurses to come in and start the IV. Next came Dr. Salinas, the anesthesiologist to check on me and let me know he would be back shortly to get me.

About, 35-45 minutes later it was my turn; I transferred onto a gurney and was given the medicine to put me under. Dr. Alvarez came out and talked to my mom as soon as the surgery was over and let her know everything went perfect. The next thing I remember was being back in my room and waking up from surgery a couple hours later. Pretty soon Dr. Alvarez was in checking on me, as well as Dr. Gabe, Dr. Rosales and Dr. Salinas though out the rest of the afternoon.

By now Jessica was there helping to translate for us when the nurses came by to take my blood pressure and give me more meds in my IV, she was wonderful too. She offered to take my mom to a restaurant for dinner. Dr. Alvarez and Dr. Rosales came by one more time before the evening was over. Then Jesus, the night nurse, helped us again if we needed translations.

The next day all of the doctors, including Dr. Alvarez, came in and checked on me multiple times. I tried to walk as much as I could up and down the halls. I was dealing with nausea so I kept making short trips around the halls (but it really helps with getting the gas they put in you out. I was also allowed to start having ice chips and that was wonderful.

The third day was discharge day and we were ready to head out. Rosy picked us up and we were on our way to the border crossing. She asked us for our passports, since you need them, to re-enter the US. Going into Mexico they didn't ask for them. Everything went very smoothly and we were on our way back to San Antonio.

We stopped about half way there for a chance to stretch and get something to drink. Finally, we were back at the hotel in San Antonio and Rosy was checking us into the hotel. I got up to my room and slept. That evening I let Dr. Alvarez and Susan know I was feeling better. Susan even called to check on me as well.

The next day was my day to travel home; our flight did not leave until the evening so Rosy arranged for late checkout. (THANK YOU ROSY!!)

Now started the beginning to the rest of my life. Dr. Alvarez has given me this amazing tool; he always says it is a tool. It's not going to do the work for you, you have to put in the hard work, too, if you want to be successful with it & exercise is key. The good thing is you can be successful. There are 4 stages to the Post-op diet, over the next 5 weeks Dr. Alvarez e-mailed me to remind me each time the next stage was happening, he sent out a reminder of what kinds of foods we could begin to try slowly. He was also checking in to see how we were doing and answer any questions we may have.

Since my surgery I have continued to listen to Dr. Alvarez's weekly radio talk show for continued support and guidance. (*NOTE: Dr. Alvarez is no longer doing a weekly radio show. He found it was easier for patients to get their answers by watching his You tube videos so he is spending a lot of time creating new videos*).

His compassion for this community is wonderful and I look forward each week to learning something new or gaining a new perspective on my journey. One of the most important parts of this journey is fitness. I swim a mile 4 -5 times a week. This has had a big impact on my success. Without it I would not be where I am today, just a little over 8 month since surgery and 10 month since I started my pre-op diet and I have lost 155 lbs. I am off my blood pressure medicines and no longer have sleep apnea.

He is an amazing and talented surgeon, with a deep knowledge about Bariatrics and a thirst to continue to learn the latest technology out there in order to help his patients be successful. Now, like many of you, I had done my research. I read all his reviews, and couldn't find a single negative comment about his practice. What you read about him is exactly what you get; we all have the same experience. I would recommend the VSG procedure with Dr. Alvarez to anyone who wants to change their life. He gives you the tool you need. YOU WILL NOT REGRET IT... I think he is the best!!

# DIET OBSESSED MOM

**Heather D.** - I am an RN from Nova Scotia Canada.

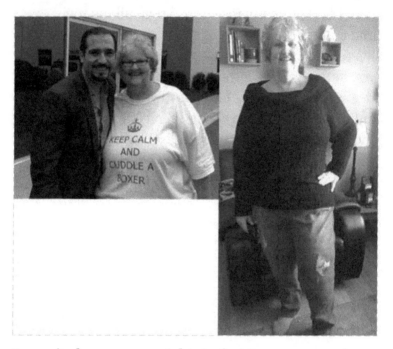

I wasn't always overweight; in fact I was a normal sized child and an underweight teenager. The problem started with a mom obsessed with weight loss and dieting that I followed with her. I believe that is where an unhealthy obsession with food began because I was literally starving as a 5'8" woman at 95lbs through high school.

After marriage and children I gained weight but high levels of activity kept me healthy and curvy but not obese. In 1994 my left knee starting causing pain and with each year mobility worsened. As I could move less and less weight came on. I was wait listed for a knee replacement and the weight gain continued.

I considered weight loss surgery on and off over the years but I did not like the idea of a Lap Band or a Bypass. I had seen lack of success for both options. Then in the summer of 2013 I discovered Dr. Alvarez and his Vertical Gastric Sleeve surgery.

I read, researched, talked to his patients, joined the Facebook group, watched videos and decided to take the plunge and head to Mexico for surgery.

My family was not 100% supportive. They were unsure of the risk I'd be taking going to Mexico and no one was able to come with me. I decided despite it all to have the surgery and contacted Susan George.

The process from there was quick and smooth. The date was set and within a few weeks I started the liquid diet that turned out to be very tolerable and I felt fine while on it.

I arrived in San Antonio the day before surgery and stayed at the hotel overnight. The next morning I met my sleeve sister, a fellow patient having surgery the same time as I was. What was funny was that she and her husband were both Nurses. All three of us RN's there at the same time to give each other support.

I met Dr. Alvarez and after some blood work and an X-ray I was set up in a room to prepare for surgery. I remember being given the shot to relax me, and apparently I was very funny following it, and the next thing I knew I was awake in my room. There was some discomfort the first 12 hours but the pain was well managed by the nurses. I was up and around within 2 hours and later in the afternoon I had a shower.

The most amazing thing to me was the care given me by the surgeons and nurses. The first day post op every hour I was checked on by a surgeon. The next day every 2 hours, and that was supposed to be their day off. I had a hernia repair as well as the sleeve but all was well. The second day I did my lots of walking to help relief the gas discomfort and the morning of day 3 I felt great and was ready to return to the hotel to start my journey back.

I returned to work 5 days after surgery and felt fine other than a little tired. I followed all the post op instructions and had a bit of discomfort because of my speed of eating and bites that were too big. Once I figured that out I was fine.

Today at almost 5 months post op I have lost 70 lbs. I feel well, have good energy, my mood is wonderful and I don't regret it for a minute. I am still waiting for that knee replacement but I know the outcome of that surgery will be so much better because of my weight loss.

I have no regret except that I didn't do it sooner, the same as most people.

I could not have had better care, and as an RN, I have very high standards. I cannot wait to lose the last 50lbs I plan to lose and know that I will be successful. I eat most of what I want, very small amounts, with the odd treat. It took about 3-4 months for the 'head cravings' to go away and for my head to catch up to my stomach. Now I cook small amounts and don't crave unhealthy things. I've found my own 'food groove' and it is working very well for me. My little secret is popsicles when I feel like I need that little something. Very low calorie, almost no carbs, fluid, and just sweet enough to fill a need.

So that's my story. When I reach my size goal, I don't focus on pounds too much, just weigh every couple of weeks. I know I can obsess and sabotage so am going by size instead. Four sizes to goal!!

# DOWN 206 POUNDS

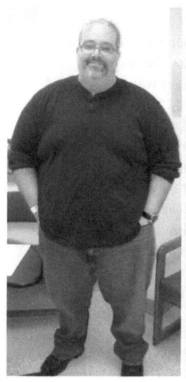 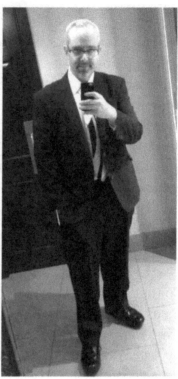

My name is Steven Simon. I am a long time supported and listener of Doc Alvarez.

When I started my research, Doctor Alvarez was the doctor I followed the closest and believed in. I actually had full coverage health insurance and my surgery was paid for here in the USA. The surgery was a success and I started losing weight the day I went on my Pre Op diet. I listen to and participate in Doc Alvarez's radio show on a weekly basis. It serves as my therapy and support group which I am forever grateful!!

My weight loss goes as follows.. April 17th 2013 I weighed 396 pounds. Today March 31st 2014 11 months later I weigh 190. Down 206 pounds in 11 and 1/2 months... I also strictly follow and subscribe to doctor Alvarez's low carb beliefs as well as exercise and participate in Martial Arts 4 days a week! I was finally able to earn my Black Belt in Goju Ryu Karate! The exam was 3 hours long and the hardest physical event of my life. I weighed 205 at that event.

The most important aspect is I'm able to play with my 6 year old son now like never before!!!

Thank god for my sleeve surgery and thank god we have doctors like Guillermo Alvarez who care about their patients and are much more than just surgeons... He believes in after care and nutrition... Most doctors just do the surgery and they don't want to know from you after!!! Thank you Doc A!!!

# FATHER DIED FROM OBESITY

**Heather D.** - I had surgery with Dr. Alvarez on December 2, 2013. I did this to save my life. My

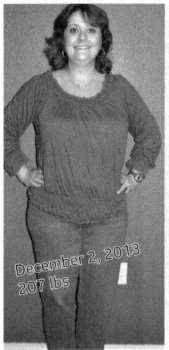
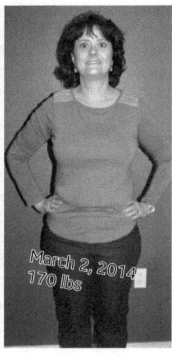

December 2, 2013
207 lbs

March 2, 2014
170 lbs

father had died the December before in 2012 from obesity and the complications it creates. He was only 65. I knew I had to do something, so I could live to see my grandkids grow up.

I wasn't "big" enough for American insurance to cover it, so I searched online. I looked at several clinics in Mexico, but all my research kept leading me back to Dr. Alvarez. I finally decided to do it.

Susan was wonderful at helping me set it up, and I flew to San Antonio alone. Susan had given me a surgery buddy who was there alone too! It worked so well that she and I had someone to share the journey with. It also reassured my husband who was at home with our children and worried that he hadn't come along.

Rosie drove us across the border and she was wonderful too. We stayed in a nice hotel and ate a wonderful homemade dinner. Then the next morning we headed to surgery. Oddly, I wasn't nervous at all after meeting Dr. Alvarez. He and his staff were so calming and wonderful. It was the best decision I have ever made. I don't regret that trip to Mexico one bit!

I am only 4 months post op, but I have attached a picture at 3 months showing 37 lbs lost. Right now I am only 25 lbs from goal weight, exercising, eating right, and feeling fabulous!

Thank you, Dr. Alvarez!

# MIDDLE AGED WEIGHT GAIN

**Nina -** I was not fat all my life. When I got married I weighed 150 pounds at 5' 9" and never gained any

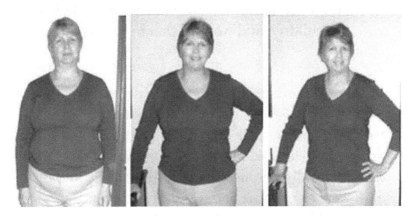

weight (except when pregnant) for the next 15 years. And then my 40's hit and I begin to put on weight until I reached my high weight of 234 pounds. I tried Weight Watchers (multiple times), Jenny Craig (multi times), HCG, Paleo, Atkins and others. They would work as long as I was 100% disciplined, but as soon as I stopped, I'd gain it back and more. My blood pressure was beginning to climb and while I didn't have any health issues, I knew it was just a matter of time.

In October 2013 I found out my cousin was going to have the Gastric Sleeve weight loss surgery. I had heard of bypass, but never had heard of the sleeve. I immediately got online and began to search to find out what it was and if it could be something for me also. I knew my insurance would not cover the surgery, so I look outside the US for a more affordable option. It was during my search for "Gastric Sleeve" that I saw the ad for Endobariatrics and followed the link to Dr. Alvarez's website and then his You Tube channel and began to watch lots of videos.

My cousin had his sleeve surgery in November at our local hospital. Final cost: $50,000 (all covered by his insurance). When I asked my cousin how many sleeve surgeries the local doctor had performed, he did not know. To me, that was an important question. I not only wanted affordable, I wanted experienced as well with a great track record for success.

During my research I found out that there were lower cost options than Dr. Alvarez in Mexico. For $4,000 I could go to a strip mall, have the surgery done by a doctor doing 11-13 surgeries that day, and then recuperate in a hotel. While I didn't want to pay $50,000 neither did I think the Walmart-type solution was best for me. I liked the idea of being in a real hospital with 24 hour nursing care with surgery performed by a doctor whose done over 6,500 of the sleeve surgeries (at that time) but not so many on a daily basis he got tired and worn out. I wanted him experienced, but fresh every day doing the surgery. I wanted him top of his game so I had the greatest chance for a successful outcome with no complications.

The clincher came when I could not find 1 person who had anything negative to say about Dr. Alvarez – and believe me, I called, chatted, and emailed lots and lots of his patients. I was even lucky enough to find a gal in my own home town who had had surgery with Dr. Alvarez and could meet with her personally. Her "before" and "after" pictures were astonishing.

Once I settled on Dr. Alvarez being the right doctor to perform the surgery, I had to decide if I was going to go through with it. Surely I could lick the weight problem by diet and exercise alone. What I haven't told you is that I had been going to a Crossfit gym for several years and was only getting bigger. If you know anything about Crossfit, you'll know it is a high intensity, hard core workout. I ate Paleo, participated in Whole 30 challenges but still saw my weight hang on.

I finally made my decision and scheduled the surgery for February 21, 2014. My husband of course knew and my cousin, but still to this day have not told our kids, my mother or any other family member. It's a personal decision, but so far I've chosen to keep it a private thing.

At the last minute, my husband could not get off work so I traveled to Mexico alone and had the surgery by myself. I'm sure some people would have said I was crazy and I'll admit I was a bit nervous. But the moment I met Dr. Alvarez in person and saw the facility, I knew I was in good hands.

Three days later I was on a plane heading home to start my new life. Surgery was on Friday and I was back to my office job on Tuesday – just 4 days later!

I have had NO complications I often read about on the online boards with people who took the low cost Mexican route or other US hospitals. I didn't know it at the time, but I've found out later that Dr. Alvarez is one of only 11 bariatric surgeons world wide with the Surgeon of Excellence designation. There are surgeons and then there are SURGEONS. Thank goodness I chose the best of the best.

I am down to 190 pounds. At age 61 I am taking it slower. Probably won't try to hit the 150 pounds mark, but will be very satisfied with the 160's. It's fun shopping my own closet to see what smaller things I can fit into next. Goodwill has become my weekly friend.

Susan, Rosey, Jessica, Anali, Dr. Alvarez and his entire surgical team are the best.

Instead of Crossfit these days, I'm kickboxing and loving it. I don't think I'll plan any marathons soon, but life is good.

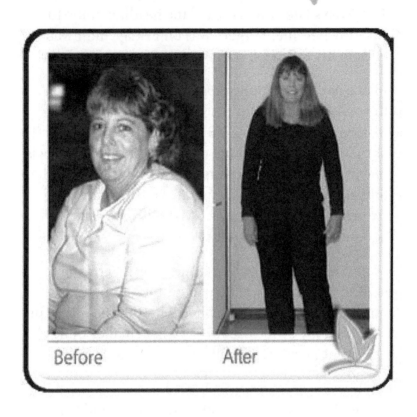

Before       After

# LAP BAND TO SLEEVE

**Susan G.** - I started on my quest for thinness about 8 yrs ago... saw a photo of myself at my BD party and was appalled at what I saw, I didn't even look like myself... 5'9 and 240.

I begin to research WLS and came across the Lapband. Unfortunately, this was right before the sleeve started to take off. I read and sought out doctors locally as opposed to going out of the country... but without luck.

I was actually told to go gain more weight and then come back and see the doctor in the US, are you kidding me?

I finally decided on a doctor in Monterrey Mexico and have my band done... I was never really happy with it, had a hard time finding anyone to do fills locally so I went back to MX a couple of times and Texas.... it was proving to be very costly... always had issues with my port.

Finally wound up with a port infection that almost killed me, had to have the band removed and heal for at least 3 months before doing the sleeve.

So that is what I did, healed.

I actually only lost 35 pounds with the band despite doing everything correctly.

The band came out and I gained back that 35 lbs so I was starting from scratch.

Finally the day came I went for my sleeve surgery and truly wondered if I was doing the right thing and almost backed out thinking... Oh I can just do Jenny Craig, or Weight Watchers one more time... boy was I thinking totally in the wrong direction, those things do not work in the long run... so I had the surgery, threw up 1 time and then there was nothing stopping me..

I really was good right out of the gate. Traveled half way across the US after surgery by car with no issues either. It took me about 8-9 months to lose my 70 lbs. I was in no hurry and I knew it was going to come off, just did what I was supposed to do and it worked.

I have maintained a 60 lb loss now for about 5.5 yrs. When you have the band, you will always be able to eat more than someone who is a "virgin" sleeve due to the stretch in the upper stomach. There isn't anything I cannot eat, portions are just smaller and I make better choices now. I also throw away a lot of food. I am physically active (zip lining, sky diving, ATV riding) and I would do it again in a heartbeat. It truly is the only thing that has ever worked for me. It is a "tool" and you do have to work with it, won't do all the work for you...you have to watch what goes in your mouth without doing all the grazing/carb eating etc. Don't know if this helps you or not, but it's my story and I am sticking to it.

# HEAVY SINCE A CHILD

**Kristen** - I am 44 years old. On 02/10/2014 I had VSG surgery with Dr. Guillermo Alvarez.

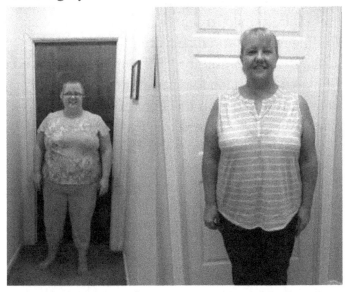

My story is similar to many I have read. I have struggled with my weight since I was a young girl. I was sad and turned to food for many years. Food was my protection – it kept people away – especially men. I did get lucky in 2008 and met a wonderful man whom I married in 2010.

In 2013, after fluctuating back and forth for many years I found myself at 335 pounds and miserable. It was time for me to take control and accept that my happiness is my responsibility. I started researching weight loss surgery.

I quickly found out that (1) my insurance would not cover anything related to weight loss and (2) I could NOT afford the 30K plus price I was quoted by my local bariatric hospital. I had heard of medical travel (or tourism) and thought maybe that was the option for me. I did hours of research. I read a lot of blogs and online forums and discovered that Mexico is rated the BEST location for VSG surgery. I gathered a list of places in Mexico for consideration. I quickly ruled out any surgeon in the Tijuana area. One primary reason why I ruled out Tijuana is some of the doctors I researched were preforming many surgeries per day, one right after another. I wanted a lot more consideration than the doctors there seemed willing to offer. Once I found Dr. Alvarez and Endobaraitric.com I thought – here it is.

The website is very thorough. I found numerous recommendations from people who had been there before. The reviews that I read for Dr. Alvarez were very encouraging. He does care.

As of 7/27/2014 I am 167 days (5.5 months) post op and I have lost exactly 100 pounds total (high weight: 335, surgery weight: 320, current weight 235). I have had zero complications and I really feel amazing. I have a long way to go but I am definitely on the right track. I have a new lease on life and I am training to do a mini marathon in October 2014. I would do it all over again in a heartbeat. I am eternally grateful to Dr. Alvarez and his staff. I love my sleeve.

# BALLOONED UP TO 258 POUNDS

My name is Teresa Crosslin and most of my life, I had

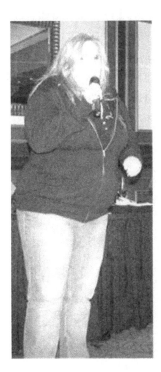
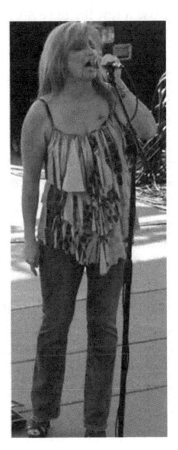

always been very thin and had always maintained a solid 130 lbs. But, after I quit smoking in Feb. 1990, I began gaining weight. Then later that year I got pregnant.

After the birth of my baby, my weight started gradually creeping up on me until I had reached what I called "the point of no return." By 2008, I had ballooned up to a whopping 258 lbs.

I had tried every diet on the market and though I would lose a few lbs here and there, I could never seem to keep it off. I would always gain back more weight than I had lost and would be so frustrated that I would just binge. Then I decided to have weight loss surgery. I searched the Internet and found Dr. Guillermo Alvarez and my life has never been the same.

It was on a Sunday afternoon and I had called the number on the website. To my surprise, It was Dr. Alvarez that answered the phone. He was very kind and answered every question of my grueling weight loss surgery interrogation that lasted for at least a good 45 minutes. By the time I had ended the call, I had no doubt where I would go for surgery.

On Dec. 2, 2008, with the support from my amazing husband and with my wonderful sister-in-law by my side, I went to see one of the most incredible and competent surgeons in the world, Dr. Guillermo Alvarez.

Dr. Alvarez had definitely put my mind at ease and I knew I was in great hands. I would like to encourage anyone who is considering having WLS, to definitely consider Dr. Alvarez and his team to take care of you. You will not find another Dr. who will care for you more than this wonderful Dr. and his great medical assistants. 5 years later and 110 lbs lost,  I have no regrets whatsoever. Thank you Dr. Alvarez, you saved my life.

# ICU NURSES BATTLE WEIGHT

**Bobby and Laurie-** surgery date 3/15/2014. It is less than a month that we are writing this testimonial but I hope it will help just one person out there that is thinking of this procedure.

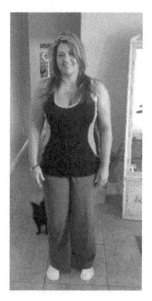
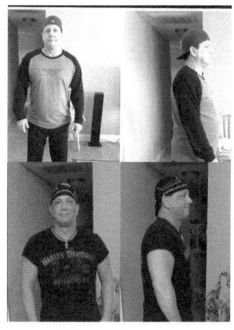

We are 49 and 47 years old respectively and our weight loss so far is 35lbs each in 21 days. We are both ICU Nurses here in Texas. We have been battling weight loss challenges most of our lives. It didn't matter what we did but the continual YO-YO dieting and night shift nursing has taken its toll on our body's.

I myself ended up at 280lbs. and suffered the last several years battling OSA(obstructive sleep apnea) and hypertension. My fiancé Laurie had also suffered from what we called "COMFORT FOODS". She was in a happier place by taking my hand in marriage and she also over indulged in those comfort foods. You don't have to be depressed to gain weight and that's why I am sharing our story.

We researched Bariatric surgery and thought we wanted the lap-band, but after two years of research and friends who had the Sleeve procedure we realized that this along with Dr. Alvarez's recommendation was the best choice for us. Now you may be thinking, hmmmm wait a minute why in the world would you go to Mexico?? I mean we are both nurses and actually know many of the surgeons and their success rates right here in Texas.

I'll tell you why, because there were nurses here that recommended him and after a long search we chose Dr. Alvarez because HE IS SIMPLY THE BEST at what he does, the Sleeve.

You have to do your research and you have to trust your gut instinct. Dr. Alvarez isn't cheap, so please don't think you're going to Mexico for a cheap surgery. We have always thought that you get what you pay for. Dr. Alvarez is so transparent in his approach and has over 265 videos on his YouTube channel. You know exactly what to expect from the moment you contact Susan--btw she is the bomb!!

Probably one of the top if not the top reason we went with Dr. Alvarez is because he does a suture(sew) line over the stapled area which reduces the chances for leaks from 3-5%(staples only) to less than 0.32%( staples + suturing).We had heard all the horror stories of Mexico but after reviewing his videos our worries were put at ease. We drove from Abilene to Eagle Pass Texas where the next day Rosie, Dr. Alvarez's cousin came and picked us up at the hotel in the Bariatric van and then drove us straight back across the border and into the hospital. This is the moment we got to meet Dr. Alvarez and his staff, btw he does surgery on Saturday as this was our day.

We knew when we sat down in the chairs of his office that this was the perfect choice for us. He explained everything in detail and answered all of our questions professionally. From this point on things move very quickly. We went to the lab and had our blood drawn. Then over to X-ray for a CXR, then back to OUR room. Yes you read that right, OUR ROOM. He provides a room with double beds for those that wish to have surgery as a couple.

Having this procedure done with your loved one gives you the best support system in the world. We were both relaxed for about 10min in our room when in comes the nurses(some speak English, but you are given a translator). They started our IV's and no more had they finished and in walks the Anesthesiologist. Incredibly nice man and excellent job of never letting us know what happened! Within two minutes the versed was in and away I went. I fell asleep right there in the room and that's where I fully woke up. 30min later my fiancé rolls in and we are together. No real pain, just pressure from the gas.

From here I must say that the hospital was old but CLEAN, the nurses are awesome and you have all the comforts of home. On day 2, we both started that stinkin thinkin, "what have we done" and "buyers remorse". It was a huge step for us not only physically but mentally as well. You have to prepare yourself to eat healthy the rest of your life. Don't be fooled by the "Oh, you did it the easy way", wrong!!!!!!

By day 3 we were back across the border and decided to stay another day as we didn't want to drive another 6 hours home. Day 4 we are home and on the Alvarez plan. Walk walk walk and more walking as the gas needs to be expelled. 3 more weeks of full liquids, then purée foods and finally back to solids.

By day 7 is the moment we realized this is not buyer's remorse because guess what folks, it really does get better. Although we are just 21 days post op and 35lbs lighter, we can feel the change. Our eating or drinking habits have permanently changed and we didn't realize for the longest that refined sugars are the devil literally. We feel more confident, outgoing and a true want to be HEALTHY. Dr. Alvarez, you and your team are amazing. God has allowed this wonderful man to give a tool to the obese people but also overweight people struggling with co-morbidities as well .Currently down 35lbs, I know longer need the cpap machine as I no longer snore. My BP is down and my fiancé has left the comfort of a Golden Corral for the comfort and health benefit of protein shakes and soups. To Dr. Alvarez, we appreciate everything you have done and have come to realize miracles happen every day. So be careful what you ask God for, cause you just might get it.

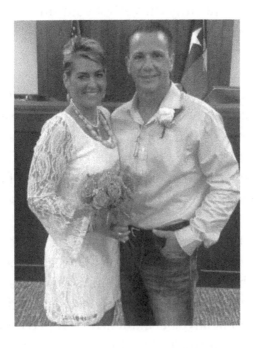

# OVERWEIGHT SINCE HIGH SCHOOL

**Holly -** Being overweight since high school and trying every diet possible was my life. After years and

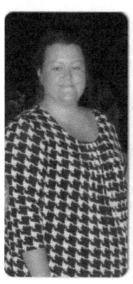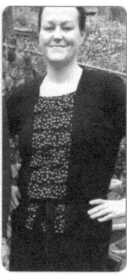

years of yo-yo dieting I started looking into the lap band but never decided on it. After having my daughter we would go visit theme parks and I never imagined I wouldn't fit on a ride. But after being told you have to get off in front of all your family really devastated me. I joined Weight Watchers and attended the meetings and was able to lose 50 pounds. Shortly after I found out I was expecting my second child. After my son was born I was able to lose about 20 pounds or so but never got serious about losing the weight. I would go to the gym and work out and try to eat healthy but never had much success. I starting looking into the lap band again, doing lots of research.

After researching night after night I came across the gastric sleeve and Dr. Alvarez. After weeks and weeks of research and speaking to a few of his patients I decided to send the email to Susan. Susan was so helpful with the whole process and made it so simple. After filling out the medical paperwork, I awaited the approval from Dr. Alvarez.

I received the email that I was a good candidate for surgery. I then scheduled my surgery. I had to do a three week liquid diet since my BMI was so high. I knew that it would be difficult but well worth it. The three weeks before surgery went by really fast. My sister n law and I drove to Eagle Pass Texas where we met the other two ladies scheduled for surgery. We all went out to eat; of course us three patients had soup. The next morning we awaited Rosy's arrival to take us across the border to the hospital. The whole process was so simple, no problems at all. Once we arrived at the hospital we each went in one by one to discuss our medical history and get our weight. I was so nervous until I stepped into Dr. Alvarez's office; he made me feel so comfortable. After visiting with him we were immediately taken to the hospital room, then on to x-ray and blood work.

Everything was so fast and smooth. Before I knew I was being wheeled out of my room to surgery and that's the last thing I remember. I remember waking up in my bed and my sister n law said I was done. I wasn't in a lot of pain, but did have some nausea. All of the nurses were so friendly and got me anything I needed. Dr. Alvarez came by every day to check on us. After our two nights we all had a short visit with Dr. Alvarez and also the nurse Jessica to go over all of the post op instructions. Rosy came to pick us up from the hospital to take us back to the hotel were we left our vehicles. I had a lot of people question my decision to go to Mexico for surgery, but this was the best decision for me. I do not regret it in any way.

I have lost a total of 135 pounds and I'm not even one year out from surgery. The best thing about it was when I was able to get on "any" ride I wanted to when we went to the theme park. To look over and see that your daughter is so happy that you can finally ride with her was priceless. I would like to say "Thank You" to Dr. Alvarez and his team. In my book they are truly "The Dream Team". They have given me my life back and I look forward to what the future holds.

# DIET AND EXERCISE WITH NO SUCCESS

I had always been thin not healthy necessarily. I graduated high school at 88lbs.

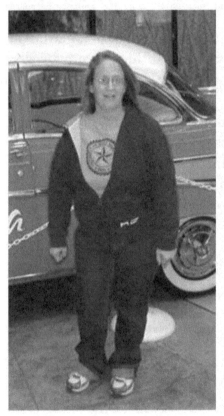
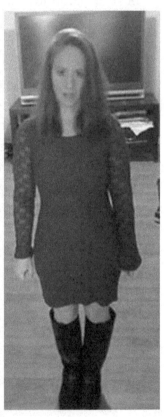

At 4 foot 9.5 inches on the bmi scale, it is a healthy weight ,but for me weight was a control thing and I suffered with bulimia all through high school. I was thin ,but not going about it the right way. I ate fast food, junk food, and rarely anything healthy. I graduated in 1992.

Fast forward to 1994 and my 1st daughter was born, people did not even know I was pregnant until around 8 months and I walked out of the hospital at 95 lbs a single parent and clueless.

I decided to go to college to make a better life for my daughter I went to a two year program and graduated one month after I had my second child in 1996.

Life was tough as a single parent with two kids so I decided to join the army (I actually was already in the us army reserves I just went active duty) and looking back this was the healthiest I had been weight wise I was around 104 and ate much healthier still a lot of fast foods due to long work hours.

Sometime in 1998 I started to have a profound fatigue and a lot of woman's issues and the army physicians did the bare minimum to help me get better. I met my husband in the army and when I got out we got married and moved to Texas this is when I started to gain weight I was pregnant with my third child in 1999 and gained a lot of weight and profound fatigue I was diagnosed with chronic fatigue and thyroid disease sometime after his birth in 2000. I did not lose the weight after he was born I still struggled with fatigue.

Life went on I probably weighed 115 to 120 which was high normal to barely overweight. At this point life goes on I was working on finishing my bachelor's degree taking care of three children, my husband got out of the military, we bought a house.

Still struggling with fatigue constantly trying to get thyroid meds right which I'm not it was ever regulated correctly. I did learn I had an autoimmune thyroid disease hashimotos and I had a goiter. I gave birth to my fourth son in 2003 and breast fed him for 17 months I thought this would help with the weight loss and it was amazing bonding experience. I worked part time at the local Walmart and took care of four kids I often got lost in the mix which was fine by me my kid were priority.

Somewhere in or near 2004 I wanted the goiter out of my body I had severe insomnia and felt it was keeping me from breathing at night so they took the goiter out and the whole thyroid gland, I felt things would improve, but I still had so much fatigue and insomnia. I guess at this rate I was gaining five lbs a year and definitely after the fourth kid was a bit overweight. I gave birth to my 5th child in 2006.

We moved to the Austin area at this point I was working full time in the social service area, and had graduated college with my bachelor's degree. The move meant a two hour commute each way and lots of fast food due to laziness and pure convenience. I slowly gained weight and would try to diet but with no success.

In 2007, I shared with my husband that my excess skin from multiple children was disturbing and affected my self-esteem I had plastic surgery to remove it and some lipo on my legs I thought this would also help with the extra weight I was thrilled with my flat stomach and began working out regularly I even had a trainer.

I maybe lost 1-2 lbs besides the surgery weight I tried weight watchers and loss 5lbs but the food became disgusting to me and working out became difficult when my commute to work became an extra hour long due to childcare arrangements. I was exhausted due to health, due to work, and eating convenience foods and drinking lots of cokes. I was probably 130 at thus point and definitely overweight. I struggled with a lot of health issues but the doctor could really find the exact cause so I was diagnosed with everything under the sun but to include chronic fatigue, degenerative disk joint disease, arthritis, thyroid disease, sleep apnea obesity, etc.

I tried shots in my back, multiple different thyroid meds , chiropractic adjustments, counseling, nsaids, sleep aids, thyroid surgery, sleep apnea surgery (tonsils, adenoids, and fixed deviated septum), plastic surgery, ect to try gain my health back and potentially lose weight. In 2008, they did breast reduction to help my back they removed 5lbs of boobs and I still had plenty left. I quit my commuting job and opened my private investigation firm cats eye in Austin in 2008 and I could work from home and be there for my kids. Sometimes in 2010, my va doc started preaching losing weight I was probably averaging 140 (about 21 lbs overweight) I was exhausted often skipped meals, drank cokes, was taking multiple medications. I had major brain fog and was just exhausted to exhausted after being a chauffeur to my kids, sports, and running my business to do anything for myself. I was put into the nutritionally supervised program I went to meetings mostly with obese, diabetic older veteran men veterans who had such amazing stories ,but were completely debilitated from their health issues(they felt helpless with the multiple issues). I struggled but I ate healthy and increased my activities still I struggled with fatigue and of course the cokes it's like liquid magic to me for some people it's a cigarette to calm them for me it's a coke.

I tried diet and exercise with no success, so my doctor got some prescription diet pills for me. It did absolutely nothing I stayed about the same. So of-course I was frustrated and dropped from the program. I tried every diet pill I saw on tv or heard on the radio without success. The diet pills that speed you up made me physically ill I tried everything. my husband mentioned wls surgery after my latest diet failure HCG drops oh my, I had lost 7lbs I was so hyped I got down to 130s ,but of course when I quit I got back quickly to the 150s (heavier then I had ever been and for my short frame this was too much, I absolutely did not look in the mirror)

I was offended when my husband mentioned wls surgery, but I visited with my mom who has become quite a bit over weight and has type 2 diabetes . I knew that I was already prediabetic based on my labs. I WILL never forget the day my doctor added obesity to my chart that was the date I knew something had to change. I just didn't know how I asked my doctor to put me back on the health program and I tried to get the veterans affairs to do the surgery even though I was obese(33 BMI) had comorbidities, but I was not a 35 bmi which is the magic number at my doctor's office. I wasn't about to gain weight to get to 35 BMI. I had lost 7 pounds and gained additional 15 pounds in a matter of six to eight or so months.

I had a friend who went to Mexico so I scoured virtual sleeve and obesity forums and found out that docs in Mexico not only do these procedures earlier they have more experience and have been doing them longer. Honestly, I had to do it but how could I afford it, I'm not proud to say but I came up with half the money from a credit card and used part of our tax return. I had many food funerals and I will say I am not proud on surgery day I was almost 160 pounds it really doesn't sound like a lot of weight right? Remember I am very short and it was enough weight to cause me many health issues I knew I needed to do something now.

I obsessed about spending the extra money on Dr Alvarez, but my husband knew that I was completely comfortable with Dr Alvarez and said "no you're comfortable with that doctor and you feel you need this then that were you will go!" And so I did, I went alone I met my surgery buddy and her mom the night before at the casino in eagle pass and we met in the lobby the next morning, the breakfast at the hotel looked good but well we couldn't indulge. Rosie picked us up and showed us a few neat things in her little Mexico town on the five minute drive to the hospital.

I want to go see this little city someday! I had been told by another patient to speak up when Dr A  said "who wants to go first?" I was terrified, alone, and just wanted to get it over with and so I was dressed, tested,  and ready to go in a matter of an hour or so it was quick. I hate iv lines and it was quick and uneventful the anesthesiologist came in and I was moved to a stretcher and I remember nothing else till I was waking up in my room. I was pretty out of it and slept off and on all day I did get up and walk circles in my room, I surfed the net a bit and rested.

I stayed awake all night though just thinking about how I did it and missing my kids and kind of reflecting on wow I went to Mexico. The nurses and doctors come in an out that day a lot I was scared and questioned what they were giving me they brought Jessica in to explain to me and then I was good I did not feel pain this day at all.

The next day they took the iv out because it was swelling my veins. I did feel pain and nauseous this day the pain was very uncomfortable but the pain pills made me nauseated so I tried it twice and quit taking them. The nurse came in when I was feeling nauseated and asked me if I felt nausea and I was afraid they were going to put my iv back in, I walked up and down the hallway looking for where I must of had surgery (never did figure it out) and surfed the net and caught up on work this day. I had ice and water this day but I hate water so I couldn't wait till grape juice on the last day.

The grape juice was the best I've ever had and I never even finished the can! My new stomach was loud! I wish I was prepared for the ride ,but it was a little rockier then I felt it wasn't so much painful as it was emotionally draining doing for myself (FIRST) and having to remind myself of my new restrictions like seriously taking the kids to the movie and not eating popcorn I did have a fruit juice bar! It's just different!  It takes time so just realize it's not a race and give yourself time to adjust you did not become overweight in one day and you won't be skinny tomorrow.

I did feel overwhelmed at first work wise, but I work for me so I could give myself time to get back to speed. Liquids was not easy for me and I still struggle there. It's a process for me. I do like my tea only now only I don't drink sweet tea well sometimes I have a half and half sweet tea just to change it up. I lost slowly and felt it was never going to happen pretty sure everyone thinks like this at some point, I struggled with what if it doesn't work, etc. lots of self-doubt.

I found the Endobaratric and virtual sleeve forums helpful the folks on the Facebook were very positive and encouraging the virtual sleeve was great for food ideas and what if this happens not all positives all the time ,but it is a resource though.

I had surgery on March 14 , 2013. I feel this is the day I took the control in my life back. I feel so much energy and in generally much better I still have issues health wise but so many things are better. I feel better I feel healthy I feel beautiful (imagine that?). I am grateful that I did go to Dr A here I am just a little over a year out and if I want to ask a question about an issue I can reach out to Dr A on social media and especially on Mondays he will answer me by name which is comforting.  I gave his book to my pcp too so I have educated her about the gastric sleeve and at my last check up she had a student doctor and she told her student she went to Mexico and had surgery and she has now added to my list of problems obesity-resolved! I know that I did this at a low BMI, to think you can fit into a category low BMI and not be Fat enough for surgery in the United States. For me it was not about waiting until I could no longer be a mom to my five kids it was about improving my quality of life so that I could be a better mom to my kids and avoid any additional health problems.

Age at surgery 39 years old, BMI 33%

Starting Weight 159.9

Today's Weight   102.8      BMI   21%

Clothing Size 12 to 1/2!

# SECLUDED IN MY OWN HOME

My journey started Nov 2012 when I decided to have surgery with Dr Alvarez. I started my liquid diet mid Jan and surgery was Feb 4th 2013.. The pics above are of me first at 347 pounds my heaviest weight (first time I'm using this photo) and the other one at 10 months post op - about 110 pounds gone. The surgery changed my life. I was almost secluded to my home and unable to do much include putting on my own boots. Today I run a little over 3 miles 5-6 times a week, plus do weights 3-4 times a week. My experience with Dr Alvarez was fantastic. I have no complaints and I have had 0 complications. I am a nurse (retired) and he is one of the finest Drs I've had the pleasure to get to know. Thank you Dr A!

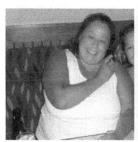 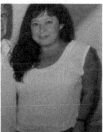 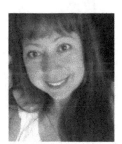

picisto.com

# OVERWEIGHT MOST OF MY LIFE

**Tobie -** Hello all let me take a minute to tell you about myself. My name is Tobie and I'm 48 years old and have been over weight most of my adult life. I'm 5'2" tall and my highest weight was 298 a lot of weight to care around. I had look into weight loss

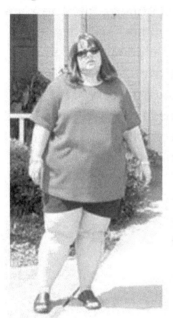
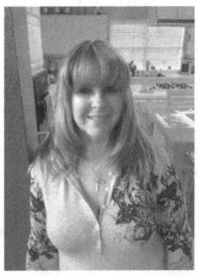

surgery for years and could never decide what to do and then I read about Dr. Guillermo Alvarez in Piedras Negras Mexico and the vertical sleeve gastrectomy (VSG). I set up a page on ObesityHelp.com and talked to people on there about the surgery and Dr. Alvarez and got nothing but great info on both. So I called Susan his patient coordinator and started the ball rolling.

I had my VSG on May 12, 2008 and have never had any regrets. I have lost one hundred and forty pounds, went from a size 3x shirt to a medium and from size 26 pants to a size 10/12. I can do many things I couldn't do before surgery like get off the floor by myself, walk upstairs without dying, cross my legs and buy clothes off the rack not at specialty shops. Here is the best reason I'm glad I had the surgery our first grandchild was born in October of 2008 and I got to be there when he was born. If I hadn't had the surgery I would never have fit in the scrubs and would have missed his birth, but because of the surgery I was able to be there for our daughter and grandson. I feel so healthy now and I'm loving life. I would do this again in a heartbeat!

Now for a little about the hospital and staff, the hospital is very clean and the rooms are pretty good size so you can bring a spouse or friend along. The hospital staff is very friendly and always right there if you need anything. I don't speak Spanish and got along just fine. As for Dr. Alvarez and his staff in my opinion there is no better. Thanks to Dr. Alvarez's knowledge and skilled hands he helped me start a new life and now it is up to me to carry on with better eating habits and an exercising program. I have my life back and it keeps getting better each and every day.

# FROM 375 TO 235 IN ONE YEAR

Hi All, My name is Danny and I had the Vertical Sleeve Gastrectomy (VSG) surgery with Dr. Alvarez on May 16th of 2010 two years after my wife Tobie had hers. To anyone out there on the fence, all I can say is this is one of the most important decisions you will ever make. I had let my weight get away from me over the years and reached my highest yet at 375lbs. On my one year anniversary of my surgery I

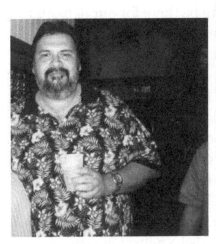
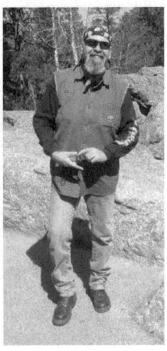

reached my goal weight of 235lbs and I have to tell you that it has been a journey like no other that I have ever experienced in my almost 50 years of life. I wish I would have taken that scary step many years before. Tobie and I researched the different surgeries and at that time we had not reached our bottom line still believing that we could lose it ourselves. We finally hit that rock bottom place in your life where nothing will stop your determination to finally lose the weight and free yourself from the everyday burdens of being overweight.

We could not have found a better Doctor than Dr. Alvarez and his staff along with the hospital personnel, they were all very professional. The hospital was super clean and the staff was very attentive.

Dr. Alvarez is one of the best in his field and is very well versed and knowledgeable, his bedside manner is so kind and caring and makes you feel so at ease and you feel like you have known him forever. He meets with you and whoever is with you and explains the whole procedure to you and then asks if you have any questions. His Nurse then takes you to get your lab work and chest x-ray, she then gets you settled into your room so you can relax until your surgery. I have to tell you I felt more comfortable with Dr. Alvarez, his staff and the hospital folks than I have ever felt with any American doctor in the states. Dr. A and his staff are total professionals. I have gotten to know Dr. A over the last almost three years, with my wife having her procedure first and then mine, Dr. A has become more than just our doctor but more as a family friend and Tobie and I both treasure that friendship very much.

Ok, about me and my journey: First visit to DR. A I weighed in at 375lbs. He placed me on a three week liquid diet (Yea I know-I won't go there). I lost 30 lbs before the surgery and had no problems, May 16, 2011 was one year for me and I weighed in at 235lbs and I'm at my goal. I have about 15 lbs of lose skin which will be taken care of in time and I should level off around 215-220lbs. 6'04 and 220lbs is my ideal weight for me. This procedure has changed our lives in so many ways to describe, Health being the biggest issue. At 375lbs I had High Blood Pressure, I was on three different medications for it, Sleep Apnea and was using a CPAC machine at night, my knees and back hurt every day. One year later and I'm off all my meds for HBP, no more CPAC machine, no more sleep apnea. I now only take over the counter vitamins (just regular one a day men's-nothing special) and feel great, my knees feel so much better, my back does not hurt, I work out three times a week and feel brand new. Dr. A and his staff will always be in our hearts.

# DEVELOPED
# ARTHRITIS AT AGE 36

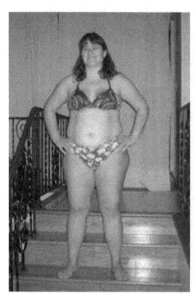 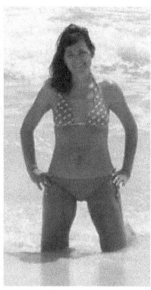

Vessela Raybosh, age at VSG surgery 37. Height:5'-2"
Date of surgery: February 17 2011
Weight before 186 lbs
Weight 10 months after surgery: 120lbs
3 years after surgery- still 120lbs
date of before picture taken 2-15-2011
date of after picture taken- April 2013

After the birth of my first child I put some weight
which I did not completely lose. After the birth of my
twins 18 months later I was definitely overweight
weighing 186lbs at 5'-2" height.
I struggled with all kinds of diets. I lost some weight.
I put double the weight several month later. At age of

36 I developed arthritis. It was painful to sit, painful to walk. I felt as if I were 60 years old. My intimate life was not exciting, I felt so old.

The best decision I made was to do the VSG with Dr. Alvarez. I did a lot of research and Dr. Alvarez had overwhelming positive feedback.

I lost my weight slow, 2lbs a week. At the beginning I was impatient and frustrated and thought I would stay overweight. But I kept losing weight and 10 months after the surgery I was 120lbs. From size 18 I went to size 0.

My life changed! No more arthritis pain. I was running up and down the stairs without being out of breath. I was running with my kids and being part of their active life. My intimate life became so much more fun. I felt not 38, I felt 28 years old. The weight loss made me feel young, look young. It made me so much more confident. I am 40 years old now and maintain 120lbs weight.

Thank you Dr. Alvarez and the whole staff! You changed my life!

# GOAL WEIGHT BY 10 MONTHS

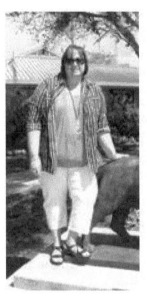 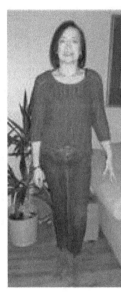

I started looking into weight loss surgery in early 2011. My weight had steadily climbed to about 275 pounds. I was starting to realize I was running out of time before I would be diagnosed with diabetes, high blood pressure or arthritis. A year after my doctor sent in the paperwork I was accepted into the Ontario Bariatric Network and began going through the process to have RNY Gastric Bypass paid for by my provincial health insurance.

Shortly after my first surgeon's visit my mother was diagnosed with terminal pancreatic cancer. I had to postpone my participation in the program to nurse my mother through her final days. After her death in November 2012 I was more determined than ever to make changes to improve my health and prolong my life.

I realized that I needed to do more research about which surgery would best fit me instead of just choosing the one that would be provided for me. I immersed myself in literature about WLS. I scoured websites, blogs and support groups to get a feel for what the different surgeries had to offer me.

When I came across Dr. Alvarez's website, read his patient testimonials and checked his credentials I had an epiphany. Strange as though it may seem I just had to find out more about his program and the vertical sleeve. I went on his YouTube site and watched every video on there. The more I did, the more certain I became that Dr. Alvarez and the vertical sleeve were the right fit for me.

On May 13, 2013 I took control of my life and I haven't looked back since. Everything connected with the surgery went smoothly. I felt like I was in great hands every step of the way. I feel that Dr. Alvarez and his team represented the surgery in an honest, straight forward manner and certainly delivered in every way possible.

I followed Dr. Alvarez's plan and am absolutely thrilled with the results. I was very "hard-core" right from the beginning and stayed with 650 calories, under 40 grams of carbohydrates, under 30 grams of fat, over 70 grams of protein and TONS of water. I began walking a few weeks out, started hitting the gym at about 2 months out and now go to aerobics, walk and lift weights 4-5 times a week.

Now that I am 11 months out from surgery I have increased my calories to about 800 most days but I am trying hard to stick with the low carb high protein regime that was so successful for me. The weight came off quite easily for the first 8 months or so with the occasional stall along the way. The last 3 months have certainly been much slower so I am really happy that I came out swinging right from surgery. I am very close to maintenance now and have started to slowly increase my calories to find my optimum range to maintain my weight loss.

I think that maintenance is the true test of any WLS. Now that I am almost there I think the real work begins. I have been able to lose the weight with the help of my sleeve but now I have to rely on the changes I have made to my diet and lifestyle to maintain it.

I was 307 lbs before surgery, 285 lbs the day of surgery, and 10 months out in March 2014 hit my goal weight of 170 lbs. I am 11 months out now and weigh 162 lbs and I am shooting for 155 lbs. That would put me in the normal BMI range for my height and at a weight I have not been for probably 30 years! I have lost 145lbs which is almost HALF of me! I worked hard to lose the weight but I honestly don't think it would have been possible without Dr. Alvarez and my sleeve! Hands down it was the best decision I have EVER made in my life! I am in control and loving it!

# OVERWEIGHT SINCE AGE 17

**Marjory** - Life is such a beautiful thing. I love and enjoy mine. However, that wasn't always the case. See, I had been overweight starting at the age of 17, which turned into obesity at 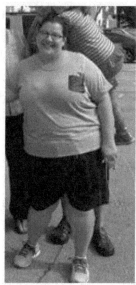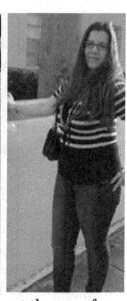 the age of 24 and then morbidly obese at the age of 34. I hated myself and cried myself to sleep almost every day, only to wake up in the morning and practice the same overeating routine, the same routine that had me in bondage for the past 17 years. I didn't know how to stop and had definitely reached a point of no return. I couldn't start and or keep a diet for longer than a few days, didn't have the energy or the desire to exercise. I just wanted to keep on with pity parties and wishing I could magically wake up one day and be fit and feel healthy. On these 17 years of pain and struggle I lost weight on my own where I was once 134 pounds only to gain it back in a period of 2.5 years. My obesity caused me sleep apnea, back and body aches, major hormonal unbalance, PCOS, depression and the list goes on. It was really hard on my family specially parents to see me this way but it wasn't easy to stop, it was a food addiction to cover up for something in my life that was rooted deep in my core. So I started to take care of myself emotionally, mentally, spiritually before I was even ready to take care of myself physically.

When I was ready, I started looking toward getting the gastric sleeve surgery to put an end to my weight issues. My sister had the Sleeve surgery by a local Dr. and she was doing great, that gave me the extra kick I needed to make my decision. Her husband helped me do some research, we looked for a way for me to have the surgery However, I did not have insurance or the funds to make that happen, which was going for about $20,000.00.

My brother in law mentioned that a lot of people were going to Mexico for the surgery. I was not against that, but it scared me a little. He kept doing more research and mentioned Dr. Guillermo Alvarez, he asked me to look him up. It took me 2 weeks' worth of daily research to come to the conclusion that Dr. Alvarez was by far the most reputable, reliable, caring and talented Bariatric Dr. out there, it so happens that he was outside the country. I saw his videos on YouTube, read plenty of wonderful, positive reviews on him and his staff, but what sold me was the YouTube video of when he did the surgery on his Mother. It was so touching to see how his mother looked at him, she was so proud of him, she was happy to see her son's accomplishments her surgery was successful and it showed.

Around the beginning of August 2013 I contacted Dr. Alvarez, spoke with his coordinator Susan, she was so pleasant and knowledgeable, I had so many thoughts, was anxious she replaced that with peace of mind. She scheduled my surgery for the middle of August; I was happy and nervous at the same time. I worked on my pre-op diet and in the blink of an eye it was my surgery date. I flew to San Antonio, then to Piedras Negras, Mexico. Luckily Susan scheduled me with the best Sleeve sister ever and since I was traveling by myself I didn't feel so lonely.
Meeting Dr. Alvarez was everything I expected and more, I had so many questions for me and he answered them promptly and my piece of mind was restored. His office was impeccable and the hospital was spacious and with all the amenities necessary for you to feel pampered (which I did). Everything was such a breeze and happened so fast, in less than 3 hours I was sleeved and without pain at all. I felt like nothing was done except there was proof on my skin that I was, he is that talented. I went home a few days later feeling amazing.

Then I began to experience the most incredible weight loss I've ever experienced, I must admit with very little effort. However, I knew that I wanted long lasting results I needed to work hard. Now I work out every day, I eat until I'm satisfied, I eat protein first. I practice all these principles now, so that they last me a lifetime. My highest weight was 245, now I weigh 157 pounds I am 30 pounds from my goal and I am confident that I will get there.

I have been given a second chance at life, a life that I love and want to live surrounded by loved ones and dear friends including Dr. Alvarez and Susan.

So I sit here today, proud and happy to tell you not to fear, having this surgery was the best decision I have ever made hands down, Dr. Alvarez was the only Dr. out there whom I felt will deliver what he promises and I was not wrong. Going to Mexico was nothing but a wakeup call that there is beauty everywhere, going outside the borders was safe and that there are people out there that were put in this world to help others and I have found two of those people in Susan and Dr. Alvarez. Thank you so much Dr. Alvarez for making my dream a reality.

# COWORKER'S SUCCESS CONVINCED ME

**My amazing journey -** It began when a coworker had this procedure done. She told me the

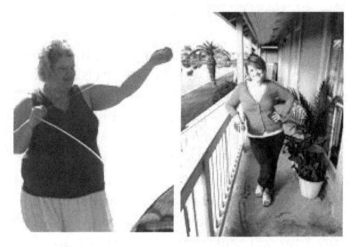

in's and outs of having any gastric operation for weight loss. As I researched our company health insurance I didn't qualify to have the operation done where I lived. I was really upset and bummed. Thinking this is it. You will die from Diabetes or Heart Disease (I didn't have either yet) I weighed over 250 pounds. I had PCOS and my gallbladder removed. Due to my PCOS I couldn't shake my weight. I actually was a runner and swimmer believe or not. My provider said I was going to have to limit the running due to the weight on my joints. I felt like I had no options.

Yet a miracle happened. I found Dr. A on believe or not on YouTube. I was researching to find any way I could do this surgery. I came across so many positive reviews of Dr. Alvarez on an Obesity website. Then I looked into his website and finally took that leap of faith. I contacted his website and received the nicest response from Susan. I explained my financials and she gave me advice. She was so patient because this really took a year for me to get my financials arranged. Now the day approached for surgery and it was like a rocket. Dr. A and Susan got me prepared of how to get there and my diet etc. Susan always encouraged me that it may be rough at first but it will be ok.

Now onto the subject of going to Mexico and having a major surgery. Yes, most people are scared. When I arrived with my husband to the clinic my nerves where settled by Dr A. I even teased him right before surgery saying "Sir I want my kidneys to stay." He laughed which made feel like it's going to be ok. My stay was there was pretty good and that was during when he was in the older hospital. Now I'm leaving out a several other crucial people. One was the personal attendant Jessica. She guided me through all of it as well. She stayed with me when I came out of anesthesia and I will admit I was emotional. A young woman who didn't even really know me sat there and rubbed my back and told me it's going to be ok. You couldn't buy that kind of customer service anywhere. Her kindness made me realize what Dr. A does is special. I also had several Surgeons checking on me constantly. They were wonderful as well and I appreciate them. To this day they check on me, which I am grateful for.

What has happened in a year's time? I have lost now 100 pounds. I have a new awareness of my body. I feel like I have been reborn and given a very special gift. I can run, jump, skip you name it. My PCOS is almost gone. I even have an old high school bathing suit from my swim team that is too big for me. I have made wonderful friends with the same surgery through this journey. I can't begin to tell you how this is a life altering gift. I truly owe my life to Dr. A and his staff. Words cannot express my gratitude.

# OVERWEIGHT CHILD

**Christy -** I have been overweight as long as I can remember. Seems like even as a child I had to watch what I ate. When my teen years came it was always

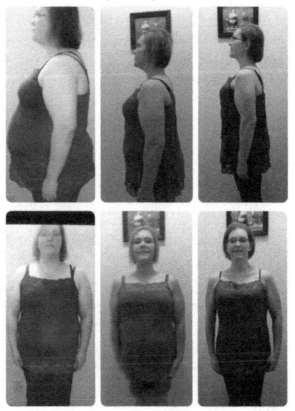

some kind of diet. Played sports in Junior High but in High School uniforms got skimpier and I felt uncomfortable because of my weight. Adulthood more dieting, diet pills, low self-esteem, and bad health. My blood pressure was high, diabetes was getting out-of-control, and cholesterol was high. I was on 3 different kinds of medication from the health problems. I was starting to have back and knee problems and not sleeping good. Years of fighting with my weight, bad health and low Self-esteem.

In 2013 I make the best decision of my life. January 17,2013 at 5'1 I was at 225 lb. Today I am off all medication and I have my self-confidence back. No more back pain or knee pain and sleeping good. I am a happy and healthy 5'1 at 136 lb on my best day and 138 lb on my bad days. I have energy now to do things with our boys. They are my world. I feel that my husband looks at me with a different light in his eye and holds me little closer. Knock on wood, I have not had any complications at all from the surgery. I know that the surgery was a tool for me to use. I work hard every day to make all the right choices.

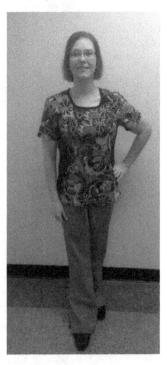

*Christy today at 137 pounds*

Dr. Alvarez and staff were awesome. Always just a call or email away. I found all of Dr. Alvarez YouTube, and Radio full of information and very helpful. I would do it all over again tomorrow. I refer anyone who ask me about my weight-loss surgery to Dr. Alvarez.

# SUCCESSFUL WEIGHT WATCHER COULDN'T KEEP IT OFF

I have struggled with my weight since I was a

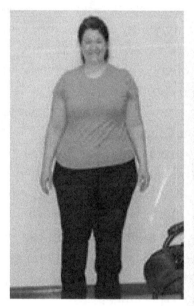
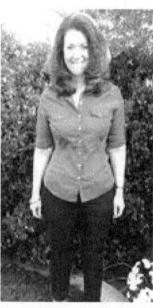

teenager. I had many successful weight losses by going to Weight Watchers. I'd lose 50-90 pounds each time (around 4 times). However, after one to two years, I would quickly re-gain the weight. In September of 2012, a very good friend of mine had gastric sleeve surgery with Dr. A. I thought she was CRAZY to have the surgery and even CRAZIER to go to Mexico. However, curiosity got the best of me and I began to research the procedure. One of the main issues I've always had is that prior to the surgery, I never felt full. No matter how much I ate. During research, it appeared that this surgery was a good answer to this and many other issues. After MONTHS of research, I learned that my insurance would cover the gastric sleeve surgery. However, they would only cover the surgery in the United States. I had come to the conclusion that I really wanted Dr. A. to do my surgery again, after thoroughly researching many, many doctors. So, I scheduled the surgery for March 28th, 2013 and my Mom accompanied me to Mexico. I was extremely well taken care of. I had no complications. I was well-informed about the pre and post issues/stages I would face. Everything went according to plan. I have lost 95 lbs. since my surgery. I am at my goal weight. I no longer have the knee pain that plagued me for YEARS. I am healthy, no longer lethargic, and have been taken off medication for my pseudo-tumor cerebre. I have no regrets and am thrilled with the outcome...and so is my doctor of 15 years. He makes sure to do the bloodwork that Dr. A. suggests every 6 months. What an amazing experience!

# GAINED 75 POUNDS IN ONE YEAR

I started my journey approximately 25 years ago. I was always a thin person until my mid to late twenties. I initially gained about 30 to 40 pounds

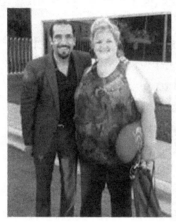
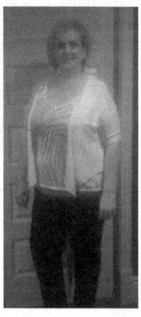

and would yo-yo back and forth for approximately 3 years and then my family experienced a tragedy with the illness and eventual loss of my father. During the last year of his illness I gained over 75 pounds. I ate my anxiety, sadness and fears away, so I thought. I was miserable and could not get control of my bad eating habits. I successfully dieted my way to 358 pounds! I tried to lose weight with every new and promising diet out there. I cannot tell you the amount of money that I spent on diets. I tried them ALL including hypnotherapy....None of them worked. My best weight loss before surgery was about 40 pounds. I would then "celebrate" and gain every pound back plus some. Last year I was DESPERATE. I was at the end of my rope. I could hardly move...I was having increasing difficulty just walking, let alone performing my duties as a nurse. I decided to look into the gastric bypass surgery. I started researching weight loss surgery on the internet and found out about the VSG. I had a consultation with a local surgeon and decided to proceed with the surgery. However, after some insurance difficulties made more complicated by the surgeon's staff I decided to look at alternatives to having the surgery done in my home state. I initially was looking for somewhere else in the US that I could have the surgery performed that would be covered by my insurance. That is when I found Dr. Alvarez. As a medical professional, I was very cautious about having surgery performed anywhere outside the US but when I found Endobariatric.com, I felt like I was personally interviewing Dr. Alvarez! His site has so much information; all of my questions were answered either by his video chats or by Susan, his coordinator.

I made the decision to have the surgery done in Mexico in May 2013. On July 17th 2013, I became a new woman!! This has been one of the BEST decisions I have ever made! I have enjoyed a 124 pound weight loss, my confidence has been restored,

I have been promoted at work and my relationships with family and friends are better than ever. I will say that the sleeve is a tool; you cannot expect it to work without you putting in work too. It is not a magic pill but it is exactly what I personally needed to be successful. I hope that someone reads my story and decides to make the decision to take back control of their lives like I did! I still have approximately 50 pounds to lose and I look forward to the journey. I can honestly say that Dr. Alvarez saved my life!

# DIETS AND BOOT CAMPS NEVER WORKED

My name is Erin. I never struggled with being overweight until after my pregnancy in 2006. I was

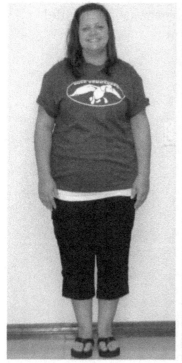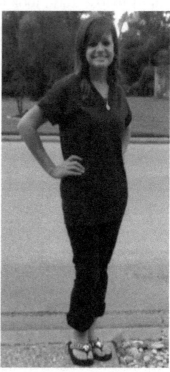

21. I only gained 25 lbs. during those 9 months and they fell off almost instantly. Over the next 7 (almost 8) years, I had put on 70 lbs. in what seemed like overnight. I would go on diets through weight loss clinics, join boot camps and even take diet pills to lose most of the weight, just to gain it all back (plus

some!) My biggest struggle was MAINTAINING. I would fall back into the same bad habits.

I went to my annual check-up with a general physician who drew lab work. My LDL levels were dangerously high (bad cholesterol) and I was headed towards diabetes at 29 years old. I knew I needed more help than I could get with surgery. I researched the internet high and low and joined 'sleeve forums' and 'weight loss surgery' groups. I read A LOT of testimonials and asked even more questions. Dr. Alvarez was the doctor who was mentioned over and over and over again. So I made the decision to go to Dr. Alvarez.

My surgery with Dr. Alvarez was on September 2, 2013. My highest weight was 220. I now weigh 117 (5' 4"). I was fortunate and had a friend go along with me and have the procedure done also.

There were no negative experiences in anything that happened before, during or after surgery. The experience that has surprised me the most, even to this day, is how fast the weight came off. I was not in pain afterwards – just uncomfortable from the gas after surgery but was definitely tolerable. No nausea.

My life has DRASTICALLY changed! Not only do I physically feel better, I am so much more happier. Even little things like being able to wrap a bath towel completely around my body, shopping for clothes in a department other than plus sizes, looking in a mirror without disgust, riding my child's toys or climbing a ladder because I don't exceed the weight limit, shaving my legs and painting my toenails has become less of a chore, smiling for a picture instead of running from the camera, dating, not consuming every single day with wondering how I'm going to lose weight and when I'm going to start doing it, hearing 'you're tiny!,' wearing a swimsuit in public, my willingness to engage in conversation with complete strangers (they seem to be much more attentive than they were when I was 103 lbs. heavier,) going to reunions/friends and family functions again because I'm not ashamed of what everyone will say about me, my energy level is sky high, I crave healthy foods instead of junk... and the list goes on!

I would recommend this surgery (most importantly Dr. Alvarez) to anyone and everyone. It will absolutely change your life, for the better!

# FELT LIKE A FAILURE

**Bethany** —Every story, every journey is a little different. I was not heavy when I was really young, but as I hit my teen years, although I managed to not be fat, the weight started to creep up slowly and then married life hit and so did the weight. Then kids, and the weight came even faster. I would work 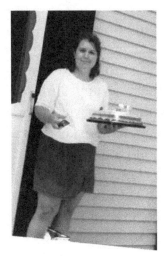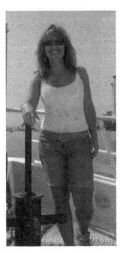 hard, I tried every diet drug, every diet. It would take 6 months to lose 10 lbs, and 3 weeks to gain that back plus another 10 because I would get so discouraged. I would work out, count every carb, every calorie, I would starve myself, and nothing seemed to work. If I did see any results at all, I usually didn't feel well, I was tired, lethargic and over all unbalanced. I hated the way I looked, I hated the way I felt, and most of all I felt like a failure, because I couldn't take the weight off.

I knew I was heavy, weight watchers wasn't working, Atkins didn't work for more than a week, and I was destroying my health with diet pills. I went white water rafting with a good friend of mine one weekend, when the trip was over, we were watching a video and slide show that the rafting company took. I was mortified at what I looked like. I had all I could do to not run out of the room crying. I decided that weekend I was going to have surgery, I wasn't sure what kind, but I knew I was going to do something.

I spent hours online researching procedures and Dr's. In 2007 the sleeve was not very common in the states. I had spent more time researching bypass &lap band. Neither was appealing to me for different reasons. I was going to do what I had to do, but neither of those procedures made me really comfortable. Then I stumbled upon an article about the sleeve, and I knew instantly that this is what I was looking for, what I needed. I researched a few different Dr's I believe I was looking at 4. 3 were in Mexico and 1 in the states. I then narrowed down to 2, Dr. Alvarez, and a Dr in Ohio I believe. I took location, and money out of the equation and looked at level of training, level of care, times the surgeon had performed the procedure, and success rate. Once I did that all signs pointed to Dr. Alvarez - a very easy, very wise decision! The level of care, the attentiveness of the nurses is far superior to anything I have ever had in the states!

I had surgery Oct 18, 2007. The day I was sleeved I was 231 pounds.

I was fortunate not to have a lot of pain with surgery, but I was unfortunate to have severe nausea and vomiting. It is a side effect of the anesthesia and it would not have mattered who did the surgery. I remember the first couple hours, it was horrible. My husband was nervous, and said out loud, we choose this, oh no we choose this. Dr Alvarez came in and mentioned that he had given me all the anti-nausea meds he could, and I remember his calm reassuring voice just saying " I know it is hard, and I can not explain it, but this will stop in the morning, when the sun comes back up. " He was right. Sometime shortly after the sun came up the vomiting stopped and I felt pretty good. I was sore, but that seemed to be more from the vomiting than anything else. I was walking the hallways and ready to go. I had surgery Thursday afternoon, and was in the van with Rosie, heading back to San Antonio by 8 am Saturday morning. Saturday afternoon John & I spent the day walking the Riverwalk, Sunday we spent watching all the shows at Seaworld. I flew back home on Monday. No one had known where we went or what we went for, and when I got back they had no idea I had just had major surgery.

So many great things have happened for me since the sleeve, but the biggest difference is how I feel about myself, I no longer feel like a failure, I no longer hide behind large sweatshirts, and fat jokes that I made about myself so that no one else had to. My self-confidence is better than it has ever been. I feel great inside and out. Losing weight has allowed me to become the person I have always wanted to be. There are people who completely love themselves and achieve great things even when they are heavy, (these people deserve a round of applause for completely accepting themselves) I was not one of those people. Now, almost 7 years after surgery is my time to wear tall shoes, tuck in my shirts, wear flashy belts, accomplish great things, and own every day!

Anyone who chooses Dr. Alvarez as their doctor has chosen someone who cares about you, about your results, he wants to know how you are doing a week later, a year later, even 7 years later. I have had health questions that even this far out I have asked Dr. A and he always answered and got right back to me. There is not a Doctor I trust or admire more. Working with Susan is like working with your best friend, she will walk you through every step, no question is silly, she knows your fears are real and she will do everything in her power to help you through them. You are not a patient at Endobariatric, you are part of a family.

My lowest after the sleeve was 142, but my body seems to be most comfortable between 148-150. I lost 89, but have managed to maintain for 6 years an 80-83 lb weight loss.

# SINGLE MOM LOSES 232 POUNDS

**Shellee** - I suddenly became a single mom of 3 kids without child support 16 years ago. I lost myself in

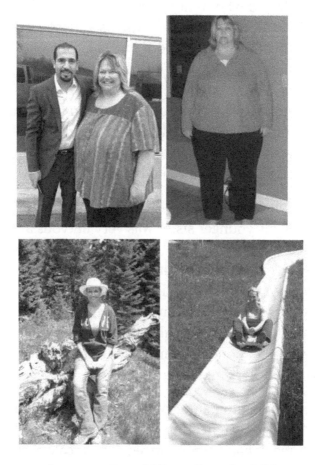

trying to take care of my kids and work. I felt betrayed and food became my best friend... and boy did it! I had my sleeve surgery January 22,

2013. One of the greatest days of my life! My highest weight was 400#. My sleeve weight was 376# and my current weight is 168#. I am 5'8" tall. I have lost 232# but have gained a whole new life!  :)

I found myself just existing. I was living to die. I was not suicidal but just numb and not living life.

I had a friend who went to Dr. Alvarez for a sleeve, so I watched all of his YouTube videos and researched everything I could find about him. The reason why I chose him is the video of one of his sleeve surgeries.  He sutured the sleeve after the stomach was removed.  The other being - I am in healthcare and could tell Dr. A was ahead of the rest of the other US surgeons and had a work ethic that spoke volumes about the man that he is.

I was planning on going alone for the surgery however my younger sister was very nervous and insisted on going with me. She was very impressed and was thrilled to share in my experience.  I had never been treated with dignity and respect as an obese person until that day... the day that I met Dr. A and all of his staff. I had also been treated with respect and kindness from Susan over the phone and throughout her emails.

I had no pain after surgery. The ONLY thing that I ever felt was a slight sting or pinching feeling where the stomach had been removed.  On a scale 1 - 10 for discomfort, a 1.  I never had any nausea although I burped a lot after surgery to get the air out of my abdomen. It was kind of funny! I burped and my surgery buddy hiccupped. My sister said it was a "gas" listening to the 2 of us! :)

My life has so drastically changed since surgery. The list of things I can do now is long!! I am hiking 5 - 5 1/2 miles 3 times a week. I am on a golf league. I work out 5 - 6 times a week. I have been white water rafting, zip lining, camping, fishing, swimming and am dating after 16 years! I have also enjoyed fair rides and riding on airplanes! I fit in the seats and feel like a normal person! I have also been alpine sliding and plan to learn how to fly fish this summer and have a snow skiing trip planned this winter which also includes snow shoeing! I am learning to do new adventures and challenge myself. I am so blessed to be alive. I am the happiest I have EVER been in life!

If I could give anyone some advice it would be to stop wasting more time! Do it! I know it sounds scary going to Mexico and not knowing what it will be like. It was the BEST decision of my life! I wish I could go again and see everyone! GREAT people and a LIFE CHANGING EXPERIENCE!!

# NO COMPLICATIONS, NO PAIN

Cindy - I am from Paragould, AR. I have been over weight most of my adult life. I have tried many diets throughout my life, which have all failed resulting in gaining the weight back plus some. As everyone

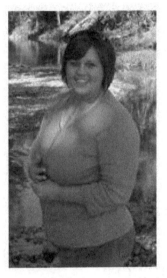 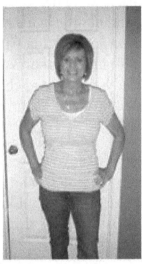

knows with being overweight there also comes many health problems. After some research I called Susan and set up an appointment to have the sleeve. Dr. Alvarez changed my life. He gave me my life back. I weighed in on the day of surgery, August 2nd, 2012. I weigh 211 lbs, wearing a size 16W jeans and 1X in shirts. I lost all my weight within the first 7 months. I now weigh 127 lbs and wear size 4 jeans and medium shirts. I have a ton of energy. No longer take prescription medicine. I have my life back thanks to Dr. Alvarez and staff. They are amazing. I would highly recommend using them to have the sleeve surgery done. It's been a wonderful journey with no complications and no pain, just a ton of weight lost.

# WEIGHT ISSUES SINCE 7 YEARS OLD

Cindy - I have had weight issues starting at 7 years old when I was diagnosed with low thyroid and

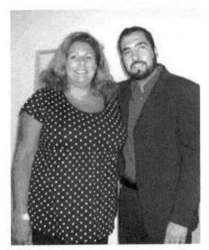
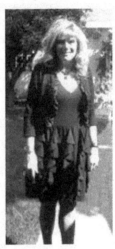

allergies including many food allergies. And let me tell you it is very difficult being a fat kid because other kids can be so cruel. By 8 years I was on the diet trail. I would lose lots of weight just to put more back on. And let me tell you, it was not like I did not try throughout my life to diet. I could tell you about almost every diet because I tried it. I was on Weight Watchers, Diet Center, The Fruit Lover diet, the Caveman's diet, the HCG Injections , liquid protein (which you had to get up the nerve every time to drink it because it was so nasty) starvation diets just to name a few. I even tried an eating disorder to lose weight. I would lose weight but then I would begin to gain it back and each time I would put on more and more. When gaining the weight I always felt so defeated and horrible about myself. It got to the point I was either starving myself or just eating everything because I was so discouraged with myself and that was not as good as the thin people.

I lived on this roller coaster till my late 40's when I finally just gave up. I reached my highest weight ever 236 pounds. I was miserable and decided to look for any other method to lose weight. I started doing research and stumbled upon lap band surgery. I even went for a consultation but it was determined that my BMI was not high enough for my health insurance to pay for the surgery. So during the time I was trying to get the decision from my insurance reversed I did lots of research online and saw all the problems that people were having with the lap band. Then someone mentioned getting the sleeve surgery. My first reaction was no way I am not getting part of my stomach cut out. But in my continued research and speaking with numerous people who had done the Gastric sleeve surgery and seeing their success without all the complications that came from other surgeries I decided that this was the surgery for me. It was my forever solution.

In all my research I found that Dr. Alvarez was a top notch surgeon. He had so many recommendations. So I go up my nerve and called Susan his coordinator. She was great in giving me all the information I needed. So I went ahead and scheduled my surgery. I was so excited and very nervous at the same time. But I knew I wanted this forever tool. I had my Vertical Gastric Sleeve surgery September 18, 2007. When we pulled up to the hospital in Mexico my stomach did a flip because I think it knew that I was leaving part of it there LOL.

I had my surgery 3 PM that afternoon. I remember Dr. Alvarez talking to me telling me Cindy it is over. You have your sleeve. I was so relieved. I slept that night (I was more tired than usual since I had not slept a whole night for about a month before my surgery due to nerves and excitement about my surgery) Then the next morning I was up walking the halls. For me I can say I had just a bit of discomfort but no real pain. Dr. Alvaraz and Susan were wonderful in the help instructions and support they provide. I continued to walk and sleep. Hospital care was outstanding. I was released from the hospital Thursday morning with medications and instructions from Dr. Alvarez. And I must say I followed ALL the instructions completely. I flew home Friday to begin my weight loss journey.

I have loved every minute of this journey. I lost a total of 75 pounds. I went from a size 22 to a size 10. And like I said before I have lost 100's of pounds in my life but this time it was different because I knew I was losing it and I could keep it off forever. Within the first year I lost my weight. And I was amazed because I was sure that I would be the only person in the world that the sleeve would not work for. I used my new tool following all recommendations and I lost the weight. I was excited and love my new body.

Now it has been over 6 years now that I have had my sleeve. And I am so happy and proud to say I have kept my weight off. I realize it is a tool, and I make good food choices and get in my fluids. I also exercise several times a week. If I do put a few extra pounds on I cut back on the carbs and lose them quite easy. I know that I will never be a fat person ever again. I know as long as I use my tool I can have the body I want.

So do I recommend the Gastric Vertical Sleeve for you? YES I do because for me it is the very best decision I have ever made in my entire life. It has made my life so much better. And after all this time there is not a day that goes by that I am not grateful for this decision and the wonderful Dr who helped me realize my dream. Would I have Dr. Alvarez my surgery if I had to do it again? Oh YES in my opinion he is the best and most caring surgeon ever. And his staff is the best. Susan is so amazing you will just love her. The only thing I regret was that this surgery was not available to me years before which would have saved me so much pain and suffering in my life. But now thanks to Dr. Alvarez I never have to endure that type of pain and suffering ever again. THANKS Dr. Alvarez I am eternally grateful!!

# CO-WORKER'S TRANSFORMATION CONVINCED HER

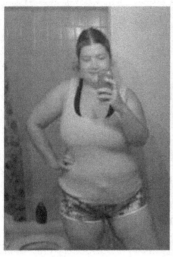

*Teisha before surgery*     *Teisha 4 months from surgery*

**Teisha -** My amazing journey. (Forgive my grammar) It began when a coworker had this procedure done. She told me the in's and outs of having any gastric operation for weight loss. As I researched our company health insurance I didn't qualify to have the operation done where I lived. I was really upset and bummed. Thinking this is it. You will die from Diabetes or Heart Disease ( Neither I had yet...) Lets back up on my health issues. I weighed over 250 pounds. I had PCOS and my gallbladder removed. Due to my PCOS I couldn't shake my weight. I actually was a runner and swimmer believe or not. My provider said I was going to have to limit the running due to the weight on my joints. I felt like I had no options.

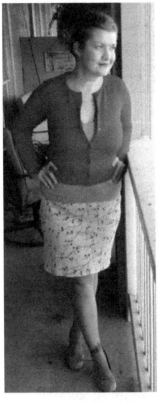

Yet a miracle happened. I found Dr. Aon - believe it or not - on YouTube. I was researching to find any way I could do this surgery. I came across so many positive reviews of Dr. Alvarez on an Obesity website. Then I looked into his website and finally took that leap of faith. I contacted his website and received the nicest response from Susan. I explained my financials and she gave me advice. She was so patient because this really took a year for me to get my financials arranged. Now the day approached for surgery and it was like a rocket. Dr. A and Susan got me prepared of how to get there and my diet etc. Susan always encouraged me that it may be rough at first but it will be ok.

Now onto the subject of going to Mexico and having a major surgery. Yes, most people are scared. When I arrived with my husband to the clinic my nerves where settled by Dr A. I even teased him right before surgery saying "Sir I want my kidneys to stay." He laughed which made feel like it's going to be ok. My stay was there was pretty good and that was during when he was in the older hospital. Now I'm leaving out a several other crucial people. One was the personal attendant Jessica. She guided me through all of it as well. She stayed with me when I came out of anesthesia and I will admit I was emotional. A young woman who didn't even really know me sat there and rubbed my back and told me it's going to be ok. You couldn't buy that kind of customer service anywhere. Her kindness made me realize what Dr. A does is special. I also had several Surgeons checking on me constantly. They were wonderful as well and I appreciate them. To this day they check on me, which I am grateful for.

What has happened in a year's time? I have lost now 100 pounds. I have a new awareness of my body. I feel like I have been reborn and given a very special gift. I can run, jump, skip you name it. My PCOS is almost gone. I even have an old high school bathing suit from my swim team that is too big for me. I have made wonderful friends with the same surgery through this journey. I can't begin to tell you how this is a life altering gift. I truly owe my life to Dr. A and his staff. Words cannot express my gratitude.

# HOURS OF RESEARCH

**Davionica** - I live in South Carolina. I had gastric sleeve surgery in Piedras Negras, Mexico with Dr.

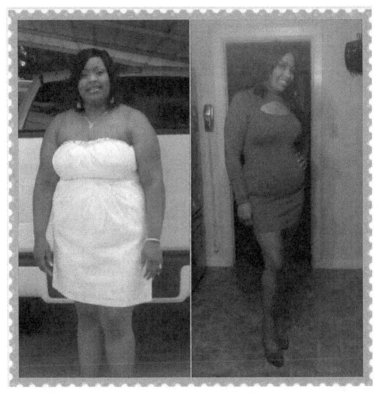

Guillermo Alvarez. My surgery date was 04/10/12. I did many, many hours of research before deciding on the surgery with Dr. Alvarez.

From my first contact with his intake coordinator, Susan, I was guided along every step of the way. Everything was thoroughly explained to me, and every question I had was answered promptly.

I flew to San Antonio where I was met by Dr. Alvarez' very nice driver, Rosy. She drove me to Eagle Pass, TX where I stayed the night. I was then picked up early the next morning and driven 5 minutes across the Mexican border to their hospital in Piedras Negras.

The hospital is immaculately clean and everyone I came in contact was completely professional and courteous and obviously knew their job well. Although I do speak some Spanish, there was never a language barrier. If someone wasn't bi-lingual, there was an interpreter by their side.

The room I was given was a spacious private room with a private bathroom. I joked that I felt like it was the "Beyonce suite at Lenox Hill Hospital in Manhattan." The room came with a desktop computer, an iPad, flat screen cable television and a couch. Even the hospital bed was extremely comfortable. And across from my room was a what I jokingly called my "Media Entertainment Center." It was a lounge with a comfy leather couch, flat screen cable TV, two desktop computers, more iPads and another private bathroom.

These accommodations would have cost a small fortune in the U.S. I made the trip with my best friend Neitra and never regretted it. She had plenty of room to sleep and entertain herself Jessica the translator also took her site seeing and to eat ant a couple of restaurants. And the entire staff goes out of their way to make sure the patient and their traveling companion are both as comfortable as possible at all times.

As for Dr. Alvarez....where do I begin? What an incredible surgeon and a wonderful human being he is. You would think that after years of performing the gastric sleeve on so many patients that he would be jaded and it would all seem so routine and boring. But not Dr. Alvarez. You can tell he has a real passion for his work, and he makes you feel as if you are his most important patient ever. My surgery turned out to be awesome I didn't have any complications at all. My family Dr. took care of all my aftercare. No complaints to this day.

One final thing I'd like to add that won't apply to everyone who reads this, but it was an important consideration for me. A state I never in my life had any intention on visiting Piedras Negras let alone having surgery there. But these concerns were all for nothing. I actually barely felt as if I was ever actually IN Texas! And although I would love to vacation in Mexico someday, I had also never been there. But I didn't feel as if I had even been to Mexico either. The hospital is literally 5 minutes across the Eagle Pass, TX border and there was a never a reason for concern as to safety or any other issue I had imagined might happen. I was treated with complete professionalism and respect by everyone, including, of course, Dr. Alvarez and his ENTIRE staff. So if you're feeling skeptical about going to see Dr. A throw caution to the wind he is amazing If I made this trip, believe me, anyone can!

# ON MEDICATION FOR HIGH BLOOD PRESSURE, HIGH CHOLESTEROL

**Thorne** - My journey with Dr. Alvarez officially started on March 6, 2013 with my emailing he and Susan requesting information about the VSG surgery. I promptly got a response and I was off and running! I had researched and talked with individuals about the surgery, but never telling anyone I was thinking about going to Mexico to have it done. I had to convince my wife that this was a good thing first!

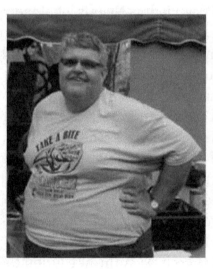 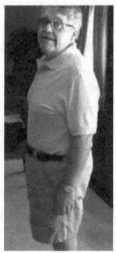

I started listening to Dr. A's radio shows on Monday at 8 p.m. and although my wife thought I was crazy for even considering going out of the country for surgery, she started listening to them with me. The education and answers to questions that he provided helped sway my wife's opinion that this was indeed the way we needed to go. That's one of the main things that impressed us both with Dr. Alvarez. He provides so much education to not only his patients but to anyone that's considering the surgery. He doesn't care if you're his patient or not, just that you have all the facts and information you need to make an informed decision.

Why was I even considering weight loss surgery? At this point, I was 412 lbs, 5'11", was on medication for high blood pressure, high cholesterol, was seeing an orthopedist about knee pain and I'd already had one heart attack and by-pass surgery and I wasn't yet 52 years old! I had been obese since I was about 7 years old and had tried every diet known to man. I'd lose 30 lbs and gain back 35. The more I researched Dr. Alvarez, the more I was convinced this was the man to do my surgery and give me back my life.

As a promise to my wife, Lorrie, I talked the surgery over with my cardiologist and my family doctor. My cardiologist and Dr. Alvarez discussed my case over the phone and through email. He was onboard. My family doctor was onboard. It was time to schedule the surgery and so now "Operation Pork Belly" was a reality! We jokingly referred my surgery as this because it was like a cooperative mission. I wasn't telling anyone until post surgery because I didn't want to hear all the negativity. My sisters and our closest friends knew, but they were the only ones. My oldest sister actually called my wife and tried to convince her this was not the thing I needed to do. I had the full support of my wife by now...sorry sis!

I started the pre-surgery liquid diet 3 weeks before my surgery date to get my BMI down from 57 and to reduce any fat on my liver. It wasn't a cake walk, but after a couple of days, I was mentally in to it. The date of surgery couldn't get her soon enough. We flew to San Antonio and then on to Eagle Pass. I was excited, but still had such a calmness about this change in my life I was making. I KNEW this was what I was supposed to do!

On Thursday, June 27, 2013, I met face to face with Dr. Alvarez. Surgery went great! I was up that night walking. The next morning still no complications. Walking the halls meeting other patients and I even went outside to the drug store next door to the hospital. I felt great! The day we flew home was the last time I took a pain pill. I took one to take any edge off that I might have for the flight and the drive home.

Since then, I've not looked back. I'm more active than I've ever been. I made friendship all over the world from having this surgery. I work in the yard, and don't have to sit down or worry that I won't be able to get up from being on the ground without someone to help me up. I just can't get over it. I walk all the time and have participated in a couple of

5k's, walking...not up to running one yet! To date, I have FOREVER lost 160 lbs!! My waist has dropped from a size 60 to a 44. My shirt size has dropped from a 4x or a size 21 to an XL or size 17 ½. I'm able to walk 5 miles or more at a time. I love my life!

I can't even begin to express the gratitude I have for the gift named Dr. Guillermo Alvarez. My life has been changed in so many ways and continues to be. As the good doctor tells us, the surgery is a tool and it's only as good as you use it. I plan on continuing to use it on the life that's been given back to me!

# IT'S NOT JUST WEIGHT LOSS

**Samantha -** I was born 10-07-1970 in Dublin, Texas. Around the age of nine I "developed early" and began to get "noticed" by men. As a way to take away the "attention" I was receiving, I consciously or subconsciously began to gain weight. It did not work as the weight gain only accentuated my development but at that point I could not stop gaining weight.

Moving ahead several years into high school... I was a good student (honors classes), had lots of friends, and did many activities within the school and the church. I was teased relentlessly about my weight (170 lbs. at 5'6") and oversized chest (36 DDD).

I worked in nursing homes or home health which was very fulfilling AND the elderly never judged me or made fun of me. I went to college on an academic scholarship and was doing really well until I was assaulted one night coming home from work. My grandmother was getting older and needed help with daily care by this time and so I left college. I stayed working in the nursing home and home health while taking care of her. It kept my mind distracted from the outside world and I felt safe once again. Occasionally I would go out when a family member would come to see grandmother.

I had an active social circle of good friends. We would get together or go out dancing. They were like a family to me but I was romantically alone. I had a boyfriend for a short time but it ended (emotionally scarring me). I became a bit reckless sexually trying to fill a void. It did not. Food became my comfort. I continued to work, eat, socialize but basically I would just "exist".

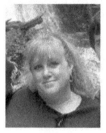

Few weeks before surgery

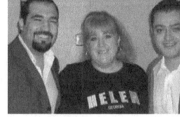

Day of Surgery

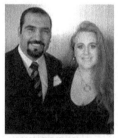

1 Year out from surgery

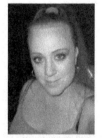

2 years out from surgery

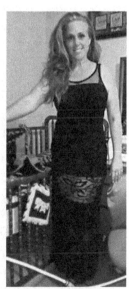

Today —5 Years Since Surgery

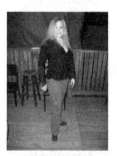

3 years out from surgery

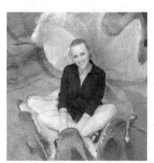

4 years out from surgery

As I got older, I continued to gain weight. At the age of 30, I decided to climb out of my emotional hole and get healthy. I moved to a new city, got a great new job, some new friends (I still have my old ones though), and a purpose... to be a new, better, healthier ME.

I was 5'7" and 210 lbs. The healthier part wasn't really hard. I ate healthy foods in small portions, exercised, and worked on my spiritual center. The only problem was that the weight was not coming off. The healthier I ate, the more weight I gained. That was NOT supposed to happen. From what I learned, working in the medical industry, I was doing everything right.

My doctor and I tried diet pills along with the healthy food. I lost a few pounds (5-10) then gained 15-20. I was baffled. Over the next few years I gained and gained and gained. How can this happen when I was doing things right? I know what you are thinking and No, my thyroid results always came back good. I was basically healthy... good cholesterol, normal blood pressure, all the lab work was normal... I was just "fat". I DID have arthritis, ADD and headaches but other than that, I was medically okay according to all the tests.

At 260 lbs., I decided to look into weight loss surgery as an option. During my research I found several "tools": Lap band, Gastric Bypass, and the Vertical Sleeve Gastrectomy (VSG). I researched for years while jumping through hoops and the red tape with the insurance company. Just when I thought I was to be approved, they changed their policy and quit covering bariatric surgery.

In 2003, I bought my first home all on my own and was starting renovating and fixing it up. I loved doing that kind of stuff--still do. Then in November of 2004 I fell on the concrete carport and injured my back, tailbone, shoulder and neck. I was in severe pain as my tailbone was dislocated and I had 1 desiccated disk with 2 bulging disks in my lower back and severe stiffness in my shoulder and neck along with the diagnosis of Degenerative Disk Disease. I pushed through the pain with medication and therapy but I was not getting any better. I hurt so bad... sitting, standing, walking, bathing, cooking, almost EVERYTHING made me hurt. After a year of the pain getting worse and becoming relentless the doctor advised me to stop working and see a specialist. I then went through a series of doctors, pain specialists and chiropractors. I had surgery to remove my tailbone (Coccyx) and was bedridden while I healed but the tailbone pain was alleviated.

Between the years 2005 and 2007, surgery worked to remove the tailbone pain but I still had the back, neck, joint and "all over" pain which caused a slew of new problems (including migraines), gained another 44 lbs., lost my job, lost my home (and most of my belongings in a foreclosure), and began to spiral downward again emotionally. The years 2007 and 2008 was, to say the least, very tough emotionally, financially and physically.

In 2009, at my highest weight (304 lbs.), I said enough is enough. I had a small settlement from a 2 year lawsuit. I took that money to pay my outstanding bills, pay back the money my family spent helping me "survive", and bought a small house. All my bills were paid and I did not owe anyone anything, being debt free for the first time ever. I had just enough money left to either put it in savings or have the VSG surgery to finally lose weight for good. I went with the healthy choice to reduce the weight in hopes of lowering the daily pain and struggling I had to endure every day.

I was blessed with a friend who gave me Dr. Alvarez's information and my life has not been the same since. I was ready --- a little scared and nervous but ready. Having gone through all my trials and hardships in the past I knew I could do this!!! After speaking with Susan and Dr. A (Alvarez) I knew I had made the right choice not only in the TYPE of procedure but in the choice of doctors. So, on May 22, 2009 I went to Piedras Negras to have surgery the following day. Everyone from Dr. A and his staff to the locals in town made my experience pleasant, memorable and remarkable! The surgery went great and I was up and around the same day with very little pain. The next day was even better and I actually drove the 4 1/2 hour trip home with my mother driving the last 30 minutes because I had become a little tired. Before I left though I was reassured that - Dr. A and his staff would still be there for me if I needed them. I thought "SURE!" --- But they have been there, every step of the way. They have treated me like family over the last 5 years and still do to this very day!!!

Over the next 6 months after surgery, I went through all the ups and downs emotionally of not really seeing much change in my body. Or so I thought!!! I was still wearing the same clothes but they WERE a little looser on me. I was going to see Dr. A in Dallas and decided to buy a new outfit. I was shocked when everything I tried on was too big and I had actually dropped down to a size 18 from a size 24. In Dallas, I was blessed with meeting Dr. Will Clower and Connie Stapleton. They have helped me along my journey as much as Dr. A has and I owe them so many thanks!!! Without their help, I would not be where I am today - --physically, mentally, spiritually, and emotionally!!! I also started several friendships with fellow "sleeve" brothers and sisters who I keep in contact with regularly. They are amazing people!!!

As everyone does, I have both struggled and thrived throughout my journey. I never reached my "mental" weight goal of what I THOUGHT I should weigh and may never reach it... But, that's okay. Each and every one is different and our bodies will decide what the "ideal" weight is and what's best for itself. My body has stopped reducing at a very healthy weight and I have maintained it for the last few years... Even though I have tried to reach my "mental" goal and have come close, my body always returns to my current weight which is just a 20 pound difference. I don't stress over it and am living life to the fullest!!!

I thank God that I had the surgery with Dr. Alvarez and his staff. I thank God I met Will and Connie because of it too. I have been truly blessed along my journey and I am happier, more centered, healthier, more confidant, and feel more alive than I ever thought possible!!! My journey isn't just about weight loss. It's about rediscovering the person I knew was hiding behind the food and under the weight. It's about healing emotionally, mentally, spiritually and physically. My journey began a LONG time ago with a young girl and choices that led to where I am today. It's been an amazing last 5 years for me and my excitement grows daily as I know that my journey is far from over!!!

# INSULIN DEPENDENT SINCE AGE 14

**Angie -** I am a mother of 3 children. A severe diabetic since the age of 14. Diagnosed with the

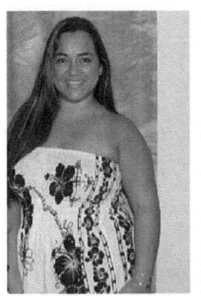
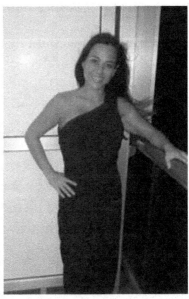

uncommon LANA 1.5 diabetes ( a bit of both types). After 19 years of medicine, finger sticks, insulin, I began to no longer care about my diabetes. Almost a depression and no regard for my condition. I started taking as much insulin needed to eat whatever I wanted. I stopped checking my glucose levels. To the point my father confronted me. Reminded me that I need to be here for my children. And at the rate I was going, I would be dead within 10-15 years.

After months of research I decided the sleeve surgery was the best decision for my health. The weight loss would be a bonus. On day 3 post-op I took my last shot of insulin. The procedure flipped a switch for me. I feel it made me stronger mentally and physically. I started off walking around the block, then 2 blocks, then 1/3 a mile, until I found myself running 5 miles.

I have completed many mud runs, challenges, and even Tough Mudder.

I play roller derby.

I have my life back!

I eat 5 to 6 small protein and produce rich meals. Very low carb. It's not a diet, it's a lifestyle. The surgery WILL not be the magic pill. It is a tool. If you use it the right way it will do some amazing things.

# CHUBBY SINCE A CHILD

**Maritere** - as long as I can remember, I was chubby. I grew up in a family where food was always a reason to gather and celebrate every and any occasion. I never heard someone telling me "stop eating", "that's enough" or "you would look better not being so fat".

At the age of 9 or 10 I remember my parents taking me to a doctor that gave me some pills for hunger (he did not say it was a diet). I would lose a little but then gain it all right back.

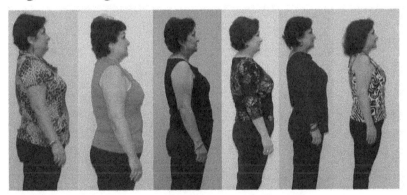

Years went by and I tried every diet that I heard about or was recommended by other people, but nothing worked. It all came back and then some.

My children saw my ongoing struggle with my weight over the years. Perhaps this was part of the reason my son decided to become a bariatric surgeon.

Now you know the rest of the story.

Dr. Alvarez is my son.

I saw patient after patient having amazing results from the sleeve surgery he performed and finally decided I wanted the surgery also.

Thank you, son, for giving me a solution to my obesity.

Thank you for encouraging me to exercise every day.

Thank you for giving me back my life.

I'll love you forever!

Mom

# ATHLETE TO 335 POUNDS

My name is Angel Ramirez Rangel, I grew up a very athletic boy playing all the sports as a young man.

In High School I was part of our Varsity Baseball and Basketball starting teams, but everything began the first year of college where you eat the same as in high school but with not the same activity or exercise. My

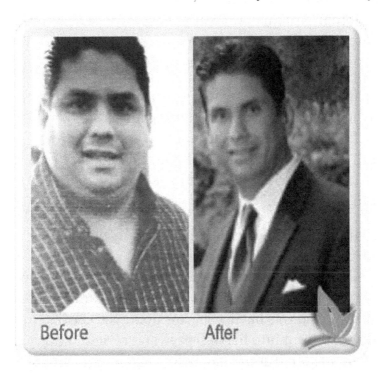

Before     After

Senior year in High School on May 1993, I was 190Lbs.

I gained 9Lbs per year to the day of my surgery on Friday October 15, 2010 when I was 335Lbs.

I had heard of the Band, the bypass and the newest surgery The Gastric Sleeve.

It was hard to decide on having the Gastric Sleeve since I had never experienced any type of surgery before, so it was difficult to accept I was overweight or to accept the BMI calculation calling me Obese and in High Health Risk.

Being 36 years old, married to my high school sweet heart Nubia and having 3 beautiful children; Arianna, Angel & Andrea. Those beautiful human beings my family were the main reason I decided to say yes to the Gastric Sleeve.

That BMI Result calling me on High health risk was a strong voice in my head bothering me day and night. I wanted to see my children grow and grow old with my beautiful wife. I had tried numerous diets and exercise and couldn't get the weight off. So Surgery it is.

Living in San Antonio and having many options of Surgeons to decide from, I was facing another challenge, who to trust my life on. I heard of a young but very good Doctor by the name of Dr. Guillermo Alvarez who was having success doing the Gastric Sleeve. I went into his web page and reviewed every single written testimonial, before and after pictures and videos of his patients.

He also clearly explains the process of the surgery and has a video of an actual surgery. The only inconvenience to me, was he was not in San Antonio but in Piedras Negras Coahuila Mexico, only a 2 hour drive from San Antonio. But he had an answer for that, he picks up his patients in San Antonio and takes them to Eagle Pass where they spend the night on a nice hotel before the surgery.

Then he takes care of transportation to the Hospital the next day and back to San Antonio after the surgery.

After Reviewing everything on his website and all those happy patients and having a much better price compared to the US, I gave the option to Dr. Alvarez. From the moment you walk into his office you can see the difference you are not in the US. The Staff treats you like person not like a dollar sign.

I met with Dr. Alvarez and he was AWESOME. He clearly explained all the questions that I had. His office the Hospital everything was very professional.

Dr Alvarez gave me his personal mobile number and all together helped me determined on scheduling my surgery and trusting him with my life. The Surgery I don't even remember, I didn't feel a thing.

I remember I was in my room and then open my eyes and said when are they taking me in, and my wife said you are back it's over.

After 24 hrs I went home and that's where the mobile number comes in handy. We talked, we Texted he was very supportive after the surgery.

I lost 151 Lbs in one year, I got under my high school senior year weight and was now at 184Lbs. Four years later the weight is off, I workout every morning, play with my kids, go on all the rides like I did this past vacation at Walt Disney World.

Dr Alvarez saved my life and I would recommend him to anyone who is in high health risk and wants a new life.

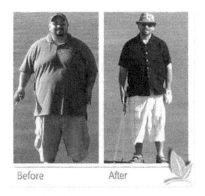

Before      After

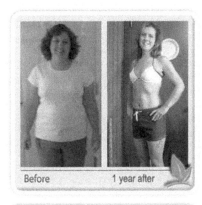

Before      1 year after

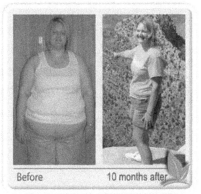

Before      10 months after

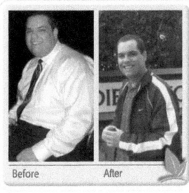

Before      After

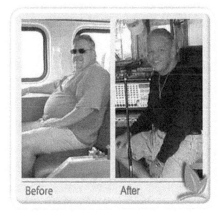

Before      After

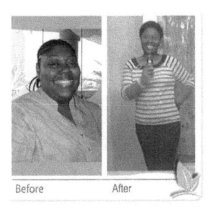

Before      After